LAUREL ALEXANDER

trotman

Nursing and
Midwifery
UNCOVERED

Nursing and Midwifery Uncovered

This second edition published in 2006 by Trotman and Company Ltd
2 The Green, Richmond, Surrey TW9 1PL

© Trotman and Company Limited 2006

First edition published in 2004 by Trotman and Company Ltd

Editorial and Publishing Team

Author Laurel Alexander
Additional material and editing Dee Pilgrim
Editorial Mina Patria, Editorial Director; Jo Jacomb, Editorial
Manager; Catherine Travers, Managing Editor; Ian Turner,
Editorial Assistant
Production Ken Ruskin, Head of Manufacturing and Logistics;
James Rudge, Production Artworker
Advertising Tom Lee, Commercial Director

Designed by XAB

British Library Cataloguing in Publication Data
A catalogue record for this book is available from the British Library

ISBN 1 84455 104 0

Typeset by Mac Style, Nafferton, East Yorkshire
Printed and bound by Creative Print and Design Group, Wales

trotman

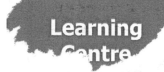
Learning
Centre

Nursing and Midwifery

UNCOVERED

Careers Uncovered guides aim to expose the truth about what it's really like to work in a particular field, containing unusual and thought-provoking facts about the profession you are interested in. Written in a lively and accessible style, *Careers Uncovered* guides explore the highs and lows of the career, along with the job opportunities and skills and qualities you will need to help you make your way forward.

Titles in this series include:

Accountancy Uncovered
Art and Design Uncovered
Charity and Voluntary Work Uncovered
E-commerce Uncovered
Journalism Uncovered
Law Uncovered
Marketing and PR Uncovered
Media Uncovered
Medicine Uncovered
Music Industry Uncovered
Nursing and Midwifery Uncovered
Performing Arts Uncovered
Sport and Fitness Uncovered
Teaching Uncovered
The Travel Industry Uncovered
Working For Yourself Uncovered

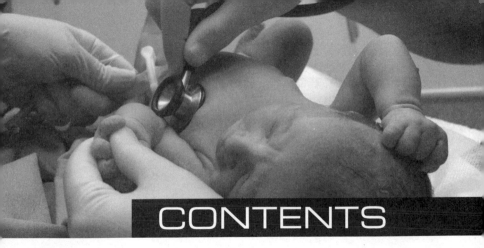

CONTENTS

About the Author

Laurel Alexander works as a complementary breast cancer care therapist with the Royal Sussex County Hospital and has a thriving private practice as a healthcare professional in Brighton. She also teaches courses in counselling skills, assertiveness training, women and health as well as being the Director of Studies for the Diploma in Holistic Stress Management, Diploma in Mind/Body Medicine and Diploma in Work-Related Stress Management, all courses accredited by the National Council of Psychotherapists. She has appeared on TV and radio giving advice on healthcare matters.

Her other books for Trotman include *Getting into Complementary Therapies*, *Getting into Healthcare Professions*, *Getting into Physiotherapy* and *Medicine Uncovered*. Laurel is also a journalist and has had health-related features published in national magazines and professional journals including *Yoga and Health*, *Positive Health*, *Reflexions* (journal of the Association of Reflexologists) and *CancerBACUP*.

Acknowledgements

I would like to thank the Armed Forces, Royal College of Nursing, Royal College of Midwives, the National Childbirth Trust, Macmillan Cancer Support, and NHS Careers for their invaluable help in writing this book. However, the biggest thank you must go to the people who are working in the nursing and midwifery sector and agreed to be interviewed: Emily Guilmant, Annie Francis, Fiona Davis, Jonathan Bradley, Terie Seignior, Sue Modeva, Maxine Holder-Critchlow, Laura Abbot and Lucy Joyce. They should all be applauded for their strength, bravery and dedication.

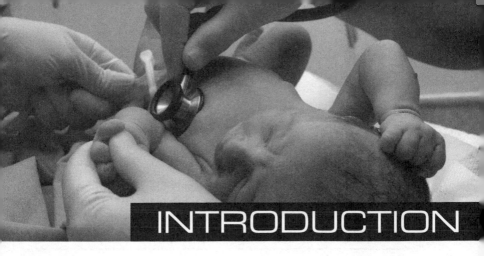

INTRODUCTION

WHAT'S THIS BOOK ABOUT?

To put it simply, this book tells you about careers in nursing and midwifery, where you could work, what you might earn and how you can become a nurse or midwife.

WHAT'S IN IT FOR YOU?

You might be looking for your first career or you might want a change of career. According to the Royal College of Nursing over 150,000 nurses in the UK are due to retire over the next ten years, so there will be plenty of opportunities for newly trained nurses to find employment. Nursing and midwifery are both fascinating careers. If you like working with people, want to make a difference to their lives in times of anxiety, and fancy being paid well for what you do then you must read the rest of this book. This chapter gives a brief overview of the sector, and finishes with a quiz to see whether you have what it takes to succeed.

MIDWIFERY

AN AGE-OLD PROFESSION

The midwife has been part of the human experience for as long as we know. The ancient Jews called her the 'wise woman', just as she is known in France as the *sage-femme* and in Germany as the *weise Frau* or *Hebamme* (mother's advisor, helper or friend). There are even two references to the midwife and her role in helping to deliver babies in the Bible.

The term 'midwife' is derived from Middle English 'midwife', or 'with-woman' (J H Aveling). The Latin term *cum-mater* and the Spanish and Portuguese term *comadre* have the same meaning: with-woman.

In ancient times the role of the midwife was not only technical but also had a spiritual or magical side. Since women had no access to formal education, it was widely assumed that the midwife's power must come from supernatural sources. The midwife had knowledge and skill in an area of life that was a mystery to most people. Hence, the midwife was sometimes revered, sometimes feared, sometimes acknowledged as a leader of the society, and sometimes tortured and killed. During the Middle Ages, several million women fell victim to a witch-burning frenzy, including midwives and healers whose power was thought to come from a pact with the devil.

MIDWIFERY TODAY

These days, midwives are seen as valued professionals and many of the women they attend in labour and birth can't praise their efforts highly enough. In fact, in the countries with the best pregnancy outcomes, midwives are the primary providers of care to pregnant women.

You could become a midwife in the NHS, based in a hospital or the community. Or you might want to be an independent midwife, working in all kinds of environments with women who want a wider range of pregnancy and labour options.

The diagram opposite shows some of the places you might find yourself working if you decide to become a midwife:

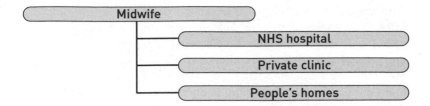

Midwife

NHS hospital

Private clinic

People's homes

NURSING

There have been huge changes in the world of nursing over the past 30 years. Where once nurses were regarded as merely low-skilled and badly paid assistants to doctors, they are now seen as valued members of our community. They have an important role to play helping our society, not only by caring for patients but also by prescribing medicines and even running their own clinics.

FASCINATING FACTS

According to *Nursing Standard* magazine, 94% of nurses are proud of what they do and would recommend becoming a nurse to other people.

One of the great things about becoming a nurse is the vast array of opportunities that open up to you once you are qualified. You could find yourself working anywhere in the world. You could be on a ward in a hospital or in a school or even a prison. How about a career in the army or RAF as a nurse? Once trained, you can also specialise and the variety of areas in which nurses work is truly mind-boggling. The four main branches are:

- Adult nursing

- Children's nursing

- Mental health nursing

- Learning disability nursing.

Within each area, you could be working in an intensive care unit (ICU), in an operating theatre, in a doctor's surgery, specialising in spinal injuries, working with the old and infirm, caring for premature babies or even treating people with tropical diseases.

Many graduates are now turning to nursing as a career. People with degrees in health or biological sciences can take a two-year postgraduate diploma to qualify as a nurse while all diploma and degree students in the UK are eligible for funding to cover tuition fees. Extra money is also available in the form of a means-tested bursary.

NURSING – A COUPLE OF KEY PLAYERS
St Camillus of Lellis (1550–1614)
St Camillus of Lellis is the patron saint of nursing. He started his career as a soldier fighting against the Turks but was forced to retire due to abscesses on his feet and his large gambling debts. These led him to gaining construction work with the Capuchin monks of Manfredonia who converted him, and in 1570 he began to live a life of penance and became a nurse at the hospital of St Giacomo in Rome. He established a following whose members took a vow to devote themselves to the material and spiritual care of the sick and those suffering from the plague. Camillus of Lellis founded the Congregation of the Servants of the Sick, and there is a hospital in Northumberland staffed by the Brothers of St Camillus.

Florence Nightingale
Born in 1820, Florence was always academically gifted and was largely educated at home by her father. On 7 February 1837, she believed that she had heard the voice of God informing her that she had a mission, but it was not until nine years later that she realised what that mission was.

She wanted to study nursing but her parents did not think it was a suitable profession. However, she made visits to the sick and she was persuaded by the then Lord Ashley to study parliamentary reports and public records relating to health matters. Within three years she was regarded by

---

influential friends as an expert on public health and hospitals. Although she went on to develop schools of nursing and played a pivotal role in transforming the way hospitals cared for the sick and injured, it is for her work during the Crimean War in 1854/55 that she is most remembered. Up until this time female nurses had never been seen in military hospitals and initially when Florence arrived with 38 nurses at the Barrack Hospital in Scutari, the doctors would not work with them. But Florence soon proved herself invaluable and she became affectionately known by her patients as 'The Lady With The Lamp'.

The diagram below shows some of the places you might find yourself working in if you become a nurse:

- **Nurse**
  - Hospital
  - A & E
  - University
  - Residential home
  - Nursing home
  - Care home
  - Children's home
  - Hospice
  - Private home
  - Women's health centre
  - Maternity unit
  - Sexual health clinic
  - Blood donor centre
  - Armed forces (army, navy, airforce)
  - Prison/secure unit
  - Pharmaceutical company
  - Cruise ship

QUIZ - DO YOU HAVE WHAT IT TAKES?

According to the Royal College of Nursing, nurses should be non-judgmental, good listeners and communicators and should empathise with people and provide support. Midwives need a similar set of skills. Answer 'yes' or 'no' to the questions listed below to see whether you might have what it takes.

- Are you a good self-manager?

- Can you be accountable for your actions?

- Do you enjoy working with people?

- Are you non-judgmental?

- Can you empathise with others?

- Have you the flexibility to juggle the needs of a number of individuals at the same time?

- Can you set people at their ease in pressurised and sometimes difficult circumstances?

- Can you be reassuring to others?

- Could you be confident at handling the distress of carers and family?

- Do you have patience?

- Have you well-developed, flexible communication skills?

- Can you cope with stressful and demanding people?

- Can you show warmth to others?

- Have you good listening skills?

- Can you provide advice and support?

- Have you understanding and intuition?

- Can you be tolerant and objective?

- Are you flexible?

- Are you reliable?

- Have you a mature and responsible attitude?

- Do you have the ability to work independently and as part of a team?

- Are you enthusiastic?

- Do you have mental and physical energy?

The more questions in the above list that you can answer 'yes' to, the more likely you are to succeed in a nursing or midwifery career.

CONCLUSION

So, do you still think you could make a success of a career in nursing or midwifery? Do you believe you've got what it takes to really care for people – many of whom will be in a distressed or frail state? If you do, then read on to discover not only what a nurse or midwife actually does – with individual patients and for the community at large – but also what a career in these two very worthwhile professions could do for you, financially, emotionally and in terms of your future career prospects.

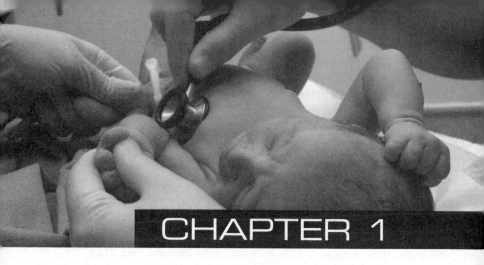

CHAPTER 1

Working in the public and private sectors

Nurses and midwives can choose to work either in the public sector, which means within the National Health Service (NHS), or within the private sector. Although the work nurses and midwives do within these two sectors is basically the same, where you work and your working hours, pay and conditions can vary. This chapter provides an analysis of each area and gives an indication of the kind of pay employees can expect to earn.

THE NHS

These days you may hear a lot of moaning about the NHS – about lack of funding, appointments that get cancelled, long waiting queues for tests and operations, patients who can't get the right treatment or the right drugs, and hospital wards that are closing. However, the fact remains that we are all fortunate to have a joined-up health service where most of our treatment is free. It's difficult to contemplate the situation that existed before the setting up of the NHS over 50 years ago when it was only those who could afford it who got medical treatment, while the vast majority had to do without.

THE SETTING UP OF THE NHS

Right up until the late 19th century the poor were discriminated against when it came to healthcare. Without the money to pay for a doctor's services or for drugs, many resorted to home remedies or relied on the charity of any well-meaning doctor who would treat them for free.

In 1828, a young surgeon named William Marsden set up The London General Institution for the Gratuitous Cure of Malignant Diseases in order to treat any destitute person who asked for help. This first philanthropical institution went on to become the Royal Free Hospital and by 1844 it was treating 30,000 patients a year. These days it is the Royal Free Hampstead NHS Trust, which has about 900 beds, and employs 4900 people treating around half a million patients each year.

However, it wasn't until the Second World War that the idea of a health service for the whole nation really started to take root. Many doctors were against it because they felt it would affect their livelihoods but they were eventually won round by the campaigning of Labour MP Aneurin Bevan. His vision was for the service to be paid for via taxation so although poorer people paid less than the wealthy in taxes (or none at all if they were unemployed), they would still benefit from the same level of healthcare. Central to Bevan's vision was the family doctor – known as a general practitioner (GP) – who could not only prescribe drugs and treatment, but could also refer people on to hospitals or specialists.

The NHS has been evolving ever since as new advances in drugs, treatments and surgery have been made, and also because the needs of the nation have changed. One of the most significant changes occurred with the passing of the NHS and Community Care Act in 1990, which recognised that more emphasis needed to be placed on services within the community rather than in hospitals, and from 1991 onwards the NHS Trusts came into being.

THE NHS TODAY

Today the NHS's key aims are:

- To promote health and prevent ill health

- To diagnose and treat injury and disease

● To care for those with long-term illnesses and disability who require NHS services.

It is the largest organisation in Europe. It is also the biggest employer in the UK, employing about 1.3 million people in England (about 5% of the population).

THE MAKE-UP OF THE NHS
The NHS consists of 633,000 professionally qualified, clinical staff, who together diagnose, treat and support patients. This includes:

● 108,000 hospital doctors and general practitioners (GPs)

● 386,000 nursing, midwifery and health visiting staff

● 122,000 scientific, therapeutic and technical staff

● 15,000 ambulance staff.

There are also 360,000 other staff, such as nursery nurses and healthcare and nursing assistants, while a further 199,000 people provide general infrastructure support in areas such as IT, catering, finance and management.

(Source: NHS)

The new millennium has seen the government pump substantial sums into the NHS after years of under-funding, and there are now new medical schools training more doctors and nurses, new hospitals and many new initiatives within the community. However, improvements have come at a high cost and many NHS Trusts have struggled to stay within their budgets. This has led to cost-cutting in certain areas, which in turn has caused unease among some sectors. In February 2006 the Royal College of Nursing issued the following press release:

'Over two-thirds (70%) of NHS nurses in the UK say their Trust is struggling with deficits. The survey of 1000 nurses also shows that deficits are hitting patient services and leading to the loss of nursing posts and job losses.

'Almost a third (31%) of nurses in the survey reported that their Trusts were deleting posts, while 66% said their Trusts were freezing posts. Over a third (38%) reported ward closures and 32% said their employer was closing patient services. More than two-thirds (69%) have seen their Trust stop the use of nurse bank and agency staff to cover shortages, and over a quarter (27%) cited that patient treatments were being delayed in order to save money.'

(Source: Courtesy of the RCN)

Sylvia Denton, President of the Royal College of Nursing, subsequently commented:

'As Trusts struggle to save money we are seeing patients suffer as services are cut and nurses are facing job losses. Crucial specialist nurses are being lost and this is unacceptable. These are nurses giving high quality individualised care. These roles allow nurses a career progression without losing direct clinical contact with patients. Keeping these posts is essential in retaining nurses within the profession. The RCN will resist attempts to make compulsory redundancies as a response to deficits. Significant progress has been made in addressing historic low staffing levels and any attempt to turn back this progress is counter productive and short-sighted.'

(Source: Courtesy of the RCN)

The debate continues.

MANAGING, MONITORING AND SETTING STANDARDS FOR THE NHS

DEPARTMENT OF HEALTH

The Department of Health sets the standards and broad working practices of the NHS and local social services. Its aim is to improve the health and well-being of people in England and so it works on ways to prevent disease and help people live longer, healthier lives. The Department of Health:

- Sets the overall strategic direction of the NHS, ensuring it is a modern health service built around the needs of patients

- Sets national standards to improve quality of services. It does this via National Service Frameworks which set out standards of care for priority areas including cancer, coronary heart disease and mental health

- Secures sufficient funds from overall government spending to ensure the NHS and social care are able to deliver these services

- Works with key partners such as the Strategic Health Authorities (SHAS), the Commission for Healthcare Audit and Improvement (CHAI) and the Commission for Social Care Inspection (CSCI) to ensure that NHS and social care organisations have the support they need to deliver the best quality care.

COMMISSION FOR HEALTHCARE AUDIT AND IMPROVEMENT (CHAI)

The Commission for Healthcare Audit and Improvement (CHAI) is an independent inspectorate and was set up in October 1999 to ensure that standards set by the Government, through its health policies and National Service Framework, are met. It also monitors the NHS to make sure it is following clinical guidance provided by the National Institute for Clinical Excellence (NICE). Local healthcare organisations in the NHS are reviewed every three or four years and if there are serious service failures then the CHAI investigates them. It also helps NHS organisations draw up action plans to tackle problems or areas of weakness.

STRATEGIC HEALTH AUTHORITIES (SHAS)

Strategic Health Authorities manage the NHS locally and are a key link between the Department of Health and the NHS. Set up in 2002 by the government, there are ten Strategic Health Authorities around the country. They develop plans to improve the health services in their own local areas, make sure the local services are performing to a high standard and increase capacity in the area so they can provide more services. Each SHA is further split into different Trusts responsible for different areas of care. The Trusts are:

- Primary Care Trusts (PCTs)

- NHS (Acute) Trusts

- Ambulance Trusts

- Care Trusts

- Mental Health Trusts.

SPECIAL HEALTH AUTHORITIES
Alongside the Strategic Health Authorities are the Special
Health Authorities which provide a health service to the whole
of England, not just to a local community. Examples are the
National Blood Authority and NHS Direct.

THE STRUCTURE OF THE NHS

The NHS provides two types of care – primary and secondary – via a
number of routes. The diagram below, taken from the NHS website,
gives an overview of how the system works, and the paragraphs that
follow explain in more detail what each care provider offers.

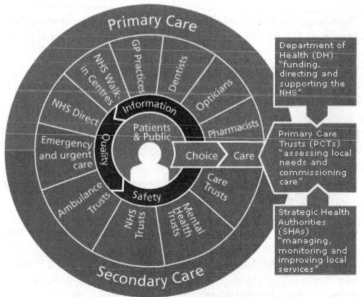

(Source: www.nhs.uk)

PRIMARY AND SECONDARY CARE

'Primary' means first – so **primary care** is basically that which is given by the first people in the NHS you approach when you have a problem. As the diagram on p. 13 shows, your primary care providers include dentists, opticians and your GP, as well as the chemist where you get prescription or over-the-counter (OTC) drugs. NHS Walk-in Centres and the extremely popular phoneline NHS Direct are also part of primary care.

If a health problem cannot be sorted out through primary care, or there is an emergency, the next stop is hospital – which provides **secondary care**. Hospitals treat conditions that normally cannot be dealt with by primary care workers and provide acute and specialist services. If you need hospital treatment, it will normally be arranged via your GP (unless, of course, it is an emergency).

PRIMARY CARE TRUSTS

Primary Care Trusts (PCTs) control 80% of the total NHS budget and so are central to its smooth operation. Because they are local organisations, they are in the best position to understand the needs of their communities. PCTs are responsible for:

● Developing an insight into the needs of their local community and assessing the health needs of all the people in their local area

● Commissioning the right services (from both primary and secondary care providers including GP practices, hospitals and dentists) to meet these needs

● Making sure these services can be accessed by everyone who needs them

● Making sure that the organisations providing these services work together effectively, including social care organisations

● Carrying out an annual assessment of GP practices in their area

● The Primary Care Trusts came on line in April 2002 and there are more than 300 of them covering all parts of England. As well as buying and monitoring services, they also play a crucial role in supporting NHS organisations. They help local GP practices, NHS

Trusts and other parts of the NHS to think more innovatively about how they can deliver better, more convenient care to their local patient communities.

NHS TRUSTS/ACUTE TRUSTS
Hospitals in the NHS provide emergency and planned hospital treatment and are managed by NHS Trusts (sometimes called Acute Trusts). These Trusts make sure that hospitals provide high-quality healthcare, and that they spend their money efficiently.

Primary Care Trusts (PCTs) purchase the services of NHS Trusts for their patients. Services include treatments where patients are admitted to hospital, day surgery which does not require an overnight hospital stay for the patient, and out-patient services where patients attend consultations and clinics.

NHS Trusts are increasingly being commissioned by PCTs to provide services in the community closer to where people live.

Most of the NHS workforce is employed by NHS Trusts: consultants, doctors, nurses, hospital dentists, pharmacists, midwives and health visitors, managers and IT specialists, as well as people doing jobs related to medicine – physiotherapists, radiographers, podiatrists, speech and language therapists, dieticians, counsellors, occupational therapists and psychologists.

There are many other support staff including receptionists, porters, cleaners, engineers, caterers and domestic and security staff who all make a key contribution to the overall experience of patients.

NHS FOUNDATION TRUSTS
The highest-performing hospitals can aspire to become Foundation Trusts, where the hospital is run by local managers, staff and members of the public. Foundation Trust status gives a hospital much more freedom in running its services than other NHS Trusts. They remain within the NHS and its framework of standards but are the new way forward as they fulfil the government's desire to see local areas become much more responsible for their own healthcare provision.

AMBULANCE TRUSTS

The NHS is responsible for providing transport so patients can get to hospital for treatment and in many areas of the country it is the Ambulance Trust that provides this service.

Until recently, there were 29 ambulances services covering England, but in July 2006, after a three-month public consultation, it was decided to merge these into 13 Ambulance Trusts.

CARE TRUSTS

Introduced in 2002, Care Trusts are set up when the NHS and Local Authorities agree to work closely together, usually where it is felt that a closer relationship between health and social care is needed. They combine both NHS responsibilities and local authority health responsibilities under a single management. This not only simplifies administration but also ensures continuity of care. This is especially true for people whose needs are more complex. For instance, an older person suffering a fall may need urgent hospital treatment, followed by a period of intermediate care to get them back on their feet, with longer-term support at home. Care Trusts aim to make the patient's journey back to health as smooth as possible by coordinating a full care package which doesn't break down between different organisations and different parts of the system. Care Trusts work in both health and social care. They carry out a range of services, including social care, mental health services and primary care services. At the moment there are only a small number of Care Trusts, though more will be set up in the future.

NHS INSTITUTE FOR INNOVATION AND IMPROVEMENT

The Institute was set up in 2005 with the express aim of raising the quality of delivery in the NHS by ensuring that improvements in healthcare delivery processes and in medical products and devices happen as quickly as possible. It has several priority programmes such as 'No Delays' (18-week wait) and 'Delivery Quality and Value'.

The best-performing organisations stand to gain more power to make decisions locally. The institute also supports NHS organisations whose services are poor or failing, by identifying problems and helping to get these organisations back on track.

MENTAL HEALTH TRUSTS

Mental Health Trusts provide specialist care for people with mental health problems. About two in every thousand people need specialist care for conditions such as severe anxiety problems or psychotic illness. This level of care is normally provided by NHS Mental Health Trusts, working in partnership with local council social services departments.

The services provided by Mental Health Trusts range from psychological therapy through to very specialist care for people with severe mental health problems.

Less complex and severe mental health problems such as depression, stress and anxiety are often treated by GPs or other primary care services and treatments might include counselling, psychological therapies, community and family support, or general health screening. With the right support and medication, many people are able to manage their mental illness themselves.

NHS DIRECT

Nowadays, before making an appointment to see their doctor for a minor ailment, many people prefer to ring the NHS Direct 24-hour phone line. NHS Direct nurses offer instant access to healthcare advice and support on self-treatment or pass the caller on to the appropriate service. If a serious condition or an emergency is reported, the nurse will give speedy advice on what to do, and may call an ambulance. You can find information and advice about the most common illnesses, and a range of treatments for them, on the NHS Direct website (www.nhsdirect.nhs.uk) or by phoning NHS Direct on 0845 4647.

NHS WALK-IN CENTRES

There are now 66 Walk-in Centres throughout England, often situated near A&E units. They provide quick and easy access to health advice and treatment for minor illnesses and injuries. You don't need to make an appointment to get seen by one of the experienced nurses who run them; you just turn up. Most are open seven days a week, from early in the morning until late in the evening, and offer a variety of services, such as:

- Assessment by an experienced NHS nurse

- Advice on how to stay healthy

- Treatment for minor illnesses such as coughs and colds and for minor injuries such as sprains or cuts

- Information on other health services such as out-of-hours care and dental services.

GENERAL PRACTITIONERS (GPS)

Most of us will, at some stage in our lives, need the services of our own GP. GPs look after the health of people in their local community and deal with a whole range of problems. They also provide health education and advice on things like smoking and diet, run clinics, give vaccinations and carry out simple surgical operations. GPs usually work with a team including nurses, health visitors and midwives, as well as other health professionals such as physiotherapists and occupational therapists. If a patient is suffering from a serious condition, or if it is beyond the GP's knowledge or expertise, he or she will refer the patient to a hospital for tests, treatment or to see a consultant with specialised knowledge. Every UK citizen has a right to be registered with a local GP, and visits to the surgery are free.

HEALTH PROMOTION ENGLAND (HPE)
Following the closure of the Health Education Authority, the HPE was established in 2000 and develops and delivers public education campaigns. It promotes healthy living by focusing on such issues as:

- **Alcohol**

- **Children and families**

- **Drugs**

- **Immunisation**

● Older people

● Sexual health.

It works in partnership with national and local organisations, both statutory and voluntary, to provide support to health and other professionals at local and community level. It is part of the NHS and works under contract to the Department of Health and the Department of Trade and Industry.

PAY IN THE NHS

In December 2004, a new pay deal for nurses known as **Agenda for Change** (AfC) was introduced, with the intention of harmonising terms and conditions for NHS workers. The system was negotiated between government health departments and the trade union UNISON, together with other health unions. However, over 18 months later it was still not in position for all nurses. Hopefully by the time you read this book, the problems will be rectified and it is expected that employers will have moved their staff onto the new pay bands, terms and conditions by the end of 2006. For more information visit www.unison.org.uk/healthcare/a4c/index.asp.

PAY FOR NURSES

Salaries vary according to your actual job description and also with the amount of experience you have. The following information is based on the Agenda for Change which, as mentioned above, has not yet been fully implemented across the country.

● **Registered nurses** (on pay band 5) earn a minimum of £19,166, and with more experience **nurse consultants** can earn up to £50,000

● **District nurses** earn around £21,630 a year if they are newly qualified, and this can rise to £34,417 for a **district nurse team manager**

● The most senior **occupational health nurses** earn around £41,242

- Salaries for **school nurses** start at around £21,630 a year for a newly qualified school nurse, to a maximum of £34,417 for a **school nurse manager**.

Nurses are also paid extra for overtime, shifts, being on-call and if they work in or near London. For example, if a nurse is on-call overnight he/she will get an extra payment of £10.46, rising to £15.61 for being on-call at the weekend and to £20.96 for a public holiday (such as Christmas or Easter). If you live on the fringes of London you get a £796 annual allowance, rising to £2844 per annum if you live in outer London and £3641 if you live in inner London.

PAY FOR MIDWIVES
Once again, salaries for midwives are determined according to job description and the amount of experience they have. Starting pay for a midwife in her first year is around £18,818 per annum but this can rise to £51,344 for a midwife consultant.

Midwives also get extra payments for overtime, shifts and calls and there is a London weighting. For example, a midwife on shift overnight earns an extra £20.45, for a weekend the payment is £27.80, and for a public holiday it is £35.49. For being on-call the extras are £10.20 for overnight, £15.23 for weekends, and £20.45 for a public holiday. The London weighting is between £825 and £1,430 if you live on the fringes, between £2750 and £3850 if you live in outer London, and between £3300 and £5500 if you live in inner London.

THE PRIVATE SECTOR

Another option is to carry out nursing or midwifery within the private sector. The diagrams opposite show some of the places you might find yourself working as a private-sector nurse or midwife.

The private sector is smaller than the NHS – but it is capitalising on customers' frustration with waiting lists, bed shortages and concerns about cleanliness in the public sector by expanding into new areas of care. Increasingly, it is also working in partnership with the NHS or (controversially) being commissioned by the NHS to provide healthcare where there is a particular capacity problem.

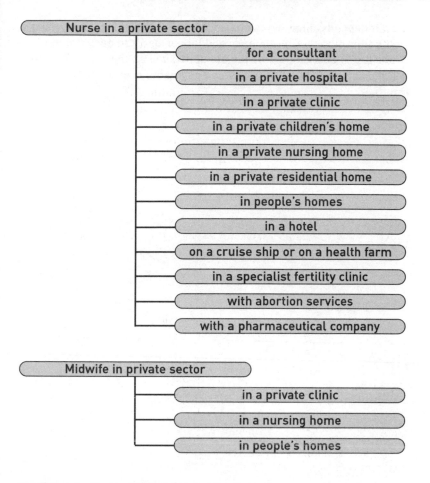

Nurse in a private sector
- for a consultant
- in a private hospital
- in a private clinic
- in a private children's home
- in a private nursing home
- in a private residential home
- in people's homes
- in a hotel
- on a cruise ship or on a health farm
- in a specialist fertility clinic
- with abortion services
- with a pharmaceutical company

Midwife in private sector
- in a private clinic
- in a nursing home
- in people's homes

PAY IN THE PRIVATE SECTOR

As a private nurse, you may be paid either by a nursing agency, which sends you out on various assignments (you could be working in an NHS hospital), or direct by the patient if you are employed by them or via the hospital or clinic you work for. You can find temporary, permanent and contract nursing work via agencies that pay between £10 and £25 per hour. Here are some examples of how much you could earn as a private nurse in central London:

● Nurse Advisor for asthma, £15 per hour

● GP Liaison Nurse, £25,000 per year.

Most independent midwives charge around £2000–£2500 for seeing women through their pregnancy and labour and can earn around G Grade (up to £30,720). Midwives are as flexible as they can afford to be, and can often arrange for staged payments over a period of time.

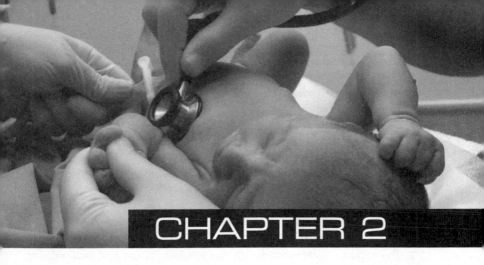

CHAPTER 2

Working for the armed forces

Earlier in this book you will have seen the many different places you can work as a nurse and one area that gives you real opportunities, both in terms of what you do and where you do it, is within the armed forces. Working in the Army, Navy or Air Force means you could be treating military personnel, their families and civilians. You could be working at a military base, in a field hospital, on a ship or even within a Ministry of Defence (MOD) hospital unit. You could be based in the UK, but you could also be working overseas, perhaps even in a war zone. Although the core training for the armed forces is similar to that within the NHS, the extra skills and disciplines you learn mean that if you decide to leave and return to civilian life both the NHS and the private sector will be very keen to have you back.

This is only one of many advantages of nursing within the armed forces, others include:

● Seeing the world ... and getting paid for it!

● Being one of a 'family' where you are part of a larger whole

- Belonging to a large and powerful institution that has tradition behind it

- Experiencing a sense of pride at serving your country.

However, you should also consider the disadvantages of nursing in the armed forces. These include:

- The dangers inherent in working in a war zone

- The nature of war wounds – bullet wounds, burns and severed limbs from explosions, even sickness caused by chemical warfare – can be extremely distressing

- Conditions can be difficult – for example in Afghanistan you could be working in sub-zero temperatures while in Iraq the heat can be stifling

- You may be expected to work above and beyond the call of duty

- You will be expected to take orders within a military environment.

Only you can decide whether this is an environment in which you'd like to work – but if it is, read on to find out the kind of jobs that are out there.

JOBS IN THE ARMY

The army is made up of two distinct areas: the regular army, which is full-time, and the Territorial Army (TA), which is part-time.

REGULAR ARMY
Personnel working in healthcare within the army are part of **Queen Alexandra's Royal Army Medical Corps** (known as the QAs). Roles within the QAs include:

HEALTHCARE ASSISTANT
No formal qualifications are required for entry as a healthcare assistant (HCA) but you do need evidence of a sound secondary education. Because they work in both MOD hospital units and in

field hospitals, HCAs receive both medical and military training and duties include:

● Feeding patients and bathing and dressing them

● Taking patients' temperatures, pulse and blood pressure

● Helping patients to use toilet facilities

● Escorting patients around the hospital.

STUDENT NURSE (WORKING IN ADULT HEALTH OR MENTAL HEALTH)

To become a student nurse with the QAs you must have five GCSEs at grade C or above including English language and a science-based subject such as chemistry or biology. However, in some cases equivalent qualifications may be considered. The course lasts for three years leading to a Diploma in Higher Education as a Registered Nurse (Adult or Mental Health). Training is both medical and military, and includes learning how to handle and maintain a weapon.

REGISTERED NURSE (ADULT HEALTH)

You must already be a registered nurse (adult) level 1 with the Nursing and Midwifery Council (NMC) or have completed your three-year student nurse course in order to become a registered nurse in the army. Many of the responsibilities will compare with those of a registered nurse working in the NHS; however, you will also receive military training and the minimum service period is four years.

NURSING OFFICER

This is really a junior management role. You must be a registered nurse (either adult or mental) level 1 with at least two years' experience in a clinical area in order to be considered for this role. Training consists of an 11-week Entry Officers Course (EOC) and a two-week professional development course. Nursing officers are expected not only to take responsibility for delivering the best possible nursing services themselves, but also to take an active role in the development of other, more junior staff members.

PAY

Soldier and officer pay depends on your rank and experience. New entrants start on £12,128.48 per annum while pay can rise to £34,310.64. A registered nurse will start at the rank of Lance Corporal with pay set at £18,294.64. Personnel within the armed forces receive subsidised food and accommodation, so your disposable income will be higher than the wage might seem to suggest.

Find out more at the Army's website, www.armyjobs.mod.uk.

TERRITORIAL ARMY (TA)

Over a quarter of the British Army is made up of part-time personnel, known as 'territorials'. That's a massive 40,000 reserve soldiers. They work alongside the regular army both in the UK and overseas in peacetime as well as in military operations. The TA Medical Services (TA MS) recruits personnel from across the healthcare sector including doctors, nurses, technicians and even students who are still undergoing their training. It runs ten independent field hospitals, two medical regiments and six medical squadrons throughout the UK. Roles in the TA MS include:

● **Healthcare assistant (HCA)** – employed in acute areas in field hospitals

● **Nurse** – make up nearly half the staff of the TA MS and are taken from a wide range of nursing disciplines.

PAY

Although TAs are part-time they receive pay that is equivalent to that of the regular army. The daily rate of pay for soldiers in the TA is £29.98 for a new entrant rising to £85.03 for a Warrant Officer, while for officers it starts at £34.31 for an Officer Cadet rising to £147.67 for a Lieutenant Colonel.

TA MSs can also qualify for 'The Bounty', which is a tax-free lump sum. In order to qualify, they must complete the minimum time commitment, which is 27 days a year if you belong to an Independent Unit, and 19 days a year if you belong to a National Unit (including an annual two-week camp). In the first year, The Bounty amounts to £371 for soldiers and officers, rising to £1462 after five years.

For more information on medical roles within the Territorial Army visit the website at www.armyjobs.mod.uk/TerritorialArmy.

FASCINATING FACTS

There are dramatic shortages of nurses in the armed forces. There is a 95% shortfall in burns and plastics nurses and a 75% shortfall in accident and emergency nurses, and there are only about half the number of nurses required for general nursing duties.

JOBS IN THE NAVY

Members of the naval medical and medical support team serve in **Queen Alexandra's Royal Naval Nursing Service (QARNNS)**. They work both in NHS hospitals and on Royal Navy bases. During peacetime they do not normally serve at sea, but at times of war they have a liability for Sea Service and serve either on hospital ships or in a medical team attached to a warship.

STUDENT NURSE
To join QARNNS as a student nurse you have to be aged between 17 and 33 years. You will need to have a minimum of five GCSEs at grade C or equivalent in academic subjects, which must include English language plus either maths or a science subject, or a BTEC National Diploma or a GNVQ Advanced level or equivalent.

STAFF NURSE
To join as a staff nurse you have to be aged between 21 and 33 years and be a RGN/RN (Registered General Nurse) on Part 1, 12, 13 or 15 of the UKCC Register. You must be recently qualified or lacking the experience to fill a junior ward sister/charge nurse post.

NURSING OFFICER
A commission as a nursing officer in QARNNS is open to RGNs who are under 39 years of age and have at least two years' post-

registration general experience in a busy hospital. Further professional qualifications are an advantage. Officers in QARNNS care for both service and civilian personnel and, as in NHS hospitals, have staff nurses and nursing students working with them.

ROYAL NAVAL NURSING SERVICE RESERVE

Alongside the regular QARNNS personnel are the **Queen Alexandra's Royal Naval Nursing Service Reserve (QARNNS)(R)**, which allows nurses to contribute to the QARNNS on a voluntary basis. They must undertake a minimum of 12 days' operational role training per year, which includes learning to man primary casualty receiving ships in crisis and war. They must also attend a number of drill nights and be available for some weekends. Reserves are also liable to compulsory call-out in a national emergency or in support of military operations and disaster relief.

PAY

Salaries start at £11,774 per annum for a student nurse for the first 26 weeks of training. After this period pay rises to £13,866. Qualified nurses start on £23,878 rising to £28,714 after a 16-week period of training on the Transition to Military Practice and the Post-Basic Professional Qualifying Course. During the course of their careers, QARNNS may have the opportunity to undertake further post-basic nursing courses in order to specialise in a particular area, such as intensive care or A&E nursing.

More information on medical careers within the Royal Navy or Royal Marines is available via the careers enquiries hotline on 0845 607 5555 or www.royal-navy.mod.uk.

CASE STUDY – NAVAL NURSE

28-year-old Jonathan Bradley is a leading naval nurse with the Queen Alexandra Royal Naval Nursing Service. He wanted to be a nurse since he was about 8 years old, and while doing a Bachelor of Nursing Adult Branch Honours degree at Southampton University he was attracted to joining the military by the pay and also the professional development.

The Royal Navy ensures you develop both as a nurse and as a military person and since joining the Navy Jonathan has undertaken a High Dependency short course, Preparation for Mentorship, Advanced Life Support, Battlefield Advanced Trauma and Life Support, ALERT course, and the IMPACT course.

"With my job in the Navy I never know where I might be," says Jonathan. "Essentially I use the skills within the NHS environment where I work. However, when I deploy I could be working anywhere and in any conditions, so these courses ensure that I can look after the military patients within the battlefield environment. Every time I go on exercise I receive updates and have my skills in patient assessment and treatment tested."

Jonathan joined the Navy in 2001, three weeks after leaving university. He went straight to HMS Raleigh where he undertook his basic training, which included everything from firing and cleaning weapons to learning to refuel ships at sea, fire fighting and damage control and even marching. The emphasis of this training was to improve his fitness and to get him to work as part of a team, while teaching him all about the Navy. After leaving HMS Raleigh he did a two-week staff nurse development course and then worked at Royal Hospital Haslar. Jonathan spent six months on a general female surgical and plastics ward and then did 18 months of surgical HDU (high dependency unit) and a year of Coronary care. During this time he was deployed for four months on the Primary Casualty Receiving Facility (PCRF) onboard RFA Argus at the start of the Gulf war in 2003, where he worked in the ten-bedded ICU (intensive care unit).

Following this he was drafted to MDHU Derriford. Since then he has spent a year on the Cardiothoracic HDU/ITU before being moved to the Acute Medical Unit (Assessment). He has subsequently completed two leadership development courses known as the Leading Rates Command Course and the Senior Rates Command Course. Both of these are compulsory promotion courses and involve learning about leadership and management of people and teams, as well as preparing candidates for promotion to the next rank. In November, Jonathan is going to the University of the West of England (UWE) in Bristol to start a postgraduate certificate.

"At present I am a staff nurse. I work in the NHS to gain skills ready for deployment. When I go to sea and am on duty it is like being on duty on a ward," he explains. "However, when off duty I am expected to be part of the ship's fire fighting and damage control team as well as completing any other tasks required by the ship – such as moving stores. The other potential operational role for me is to work with Commando Forward Surgical Group, which forms two highly mobile surgical teams that can leapfrog each other to keep a surgical facility as near to the front line as possible."

As is true with every other nurse interviewed for this book, what Jonathan likes best about what he does is the variety. "I can ask to move between specialities within the trust, if there is a space, and I can prove the operational relevance. I also get a varied year with military exercises and training as well as the potential to go on adventurous expeditions. The camaraderie of the Navy is another thing that I enjoy. There is a good team spirit and this often gets you through situations that you would otherwise be nervous about."

At the time of writing, the British Armed Forces were deployed in many countries overseas and if you are thinking about nursing in the Navy, Jonathan says this is something you must take into consideration. "There is a potential for you to be away from your family quite a lot, which can be stressful and place a strain on relationships," he says.

Jonathan now has two potential routes for him to progress in his career. He has been selected for promotion for Petty Officer Naval Nurse so he can start to develop his career in management. His second route would be to become an Officer. This would mean a return to basic training, again at

Britannia Royal Naval College, which would focus on military management rather than clinical management. In order to succeed he says you must be determined, self-disciplined and able to cope with a rank structure. "Sometimes this can be really hard as a nurse because your clinical skills do not always correlate with your rank, which can be a bit frustrating."

If you would like to learn more about nursing in the Navy or other Armed Forces you can get information from your local careers office, or from the websites quoted in this chapter. Do be aware of the need to keep fit and the fact you will be deployed to war zones potentially near the front line. Finally, Jonathan's best piece of advice for those who are keen to serve their country in this capacity is: "Be prepared to think outside of the box. As the saying goes 'be flexible, adapt and overcome!'"

JOBS IN THE AIR FORCE

Medical staff within the RAF serve in **Princess Mary's Royal Air Force Nursing Service (PMRAFNS)**. They work in NHS hospitals and on RAF bases in the UK as well as overseas.

STUDENT STAFF NURSE (RGN)
There is a three-year training course for student nurses. Entry requirements are a minimum of 200 UCAS points at Advanced level, as well as GCSEs/SCEs at grade C/3, or equivalent in English language, maths and a science-based subject. Successful graduation will lead to registration as a Registered Nurse (Adult) on the Professional Register of the Nursing and Midwifery Council (NMC), together with the award of a BSc (Hons) in Nursing. On the successful completion of the course candidates enter the service as a staff nurse (see below).

STAFF NURSE (RGN)
Registered General Nurses (RGNs) provide care not only for RAF personnel, but also for entitled civilians and personnel from other

services. Entry requirements include professional qualifications, RGN/NMC.

STAFF NURSE (RMN)

Registered Mental Nurses (RMNs) work in a team with people from many different disciplines, including psychiatry, at departments of community psychiatry. Again, entry requirements include professional qualifications – RMN/NMC. A current full driving licence is also required.

PAY

After one year, student staff nurses' pay is £16,350 per annum, while for both RGN and RMN staff nurses the pay is £24,600.

For more information about a career with the PMRAFNS visit the website www.rafcareers.com or contact the nursing liaison team on 01400 266782 / nslo@raf-careers.raf.mod.uk.

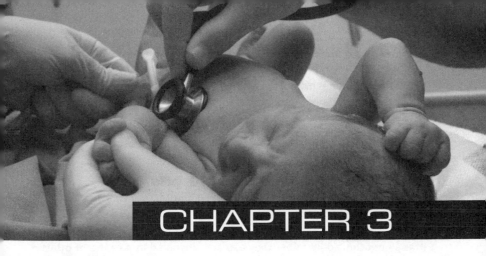

CHAPTER 3

Where nursing could take you

Becoming a nurse in the civilian world can lead to a wealth of choices as far as specialisation is concerned. Where you end up will very much depend on what your own interests are. For instance, you may wish to work with children, or to concentrate on a surgical role. You might like a role based in the community (for example being attached to a GP's surgery) or you may feel you have the qualities needed to work with patients with mental problems. This chapter explores the main areas nurses work in and outlines what they actually do there.

ACCIDENT AND EMERGENCY NURSING (A&E)

Anyone who has seen the popular American TV series *ER* will know that A&E nurses are the first port of call for people who have been in car or work accidents, or who have been taken ill suddenly. They examine everyone entering the A&E department and prioritise who should be seen first. They initiate the immediate care of patients and prescribe, initiate and monitor interventions. So in A&E you could be working with people with broken limbs, those with concussion, babies who have suddenly developed meningitis, or even those brought in with acute abdominal pain. One-third of patients seen in A&E are children, so many children's nurses work within this department (see children's nurses section, below).

BLOOD TRANSFUSION NURSING

Blood transfusion nurses assess the health and fitness of potential donors and support them through the blood donation process. But this is not their only role – they are also involved in a range of other services, such as stem cell harvesting and plasma exchange regimes.

BREAST CARE NURSING

It takes a special kind of person to fill the sensitive role of breast care nurse. At present there are around 400 breast care nurses working in the UK. They provide information, care and support in the form of counselling for women who have found a lump in their breast and need to ascertain whether it is malignant, and for women who are having treatment for breast cancer.

Some breast care nurses run their own prosthetic fitting service for women who have had mastectomies and can advise them on suitable bras and swimwear. They also educate other medical staff on the psychological care of breast cancer patients. The breast care nurse works with a large team of other people including physiotherapists, social workers and psychiatrists and some even run self-help groups for women who have survived breast cancer.

CHILDREN'S NURSING

This is one of the four main branches of nursing and covers a huge array of roles. Children's nurses work with those between 0 and 18 years old in a variety of settings, from specialist baby care units to adolescent services. Many children's nurses specialise in areas such as burns and plastics, intensive care, child protection and cancer care.

Within hospitals, children's nurses work on general and specialist in-patient wards, as well as in outpatients, intensive care and day care services. A&E departments employ children's nurses, as approximately one-third of attendees at A&E departments are children. In the independent sector there are a number of posts for children's nurses in private hospitals.

Roles for children's nurses working in the community rather than in a hospital include:

- Community children's nurse

- Practice nurse or a clinical nurse specialist (working with children with complex health needs such as diabetes and cystic fibrosis)

- School nursing service (in either the state or the private sector; many independent schools, particularly residential and boarding schools, employ a school nurse or matron).

CASE STUDY – CHILDREN'S NURSE

27-year-old Emily Guilmant is currently a Clinical Response Nurse (Band 6) at Great Ormond Street Children's Hospital in London. She always enjoyed science and interacting with children so, from 14 years old, she actively pursued finding a job that combined these interests. She did A levels in human biology, history and home economics, with a certificate in childcare, and then went to London South Bank University and gained a Diploma in Higher Education (Children's Nursing). She is currently studying part-time to gain her degree in Paediatric High Dependency Nursing.

'My GCSEs and A levels gave me a sound starting point for my nursing studies, both in the art of learning and in the knowledge itself, and my diploma allowed me to register as a children's nurse with the Nursing and Midwifery Council (NMC),' Emily explains. 'My degree is improving my working knowledge of sick children and will help with job promotion.'

Emily works long days and nights, plus weekends (11½-hour shifts). As a Clinical Response Nurse, she is part of a team that covers the whole hospital. The team supports staff caring for the sickest children on the wards, providing high-dependency nursing as well as intensive care nursing skills. Emily's work might include:

- Administering drugs that only a few nurses in the trust are able to give

- Repairing intravenous lines

- Taking blood

- Transferring sick children from the wards to intensive care (and sometimes caring for those children in intensive care units)

- Supporting nurses receiving children from intensive care. These children are still quite sick and categorised as 'high dependency'.

Out of hours, Clinical Response Nurses deal with any staffing issues that arise, and are available to answer any questions staff might have about various aspects of children's care and its delivery.

What Emily likes most about her job is the variety, because no two days are the same. 'Mostly the children make the work worthwhile, and you get to work in partnership with their family to ensure the best care', she says. However, she does have to work nights and weekends. 'This can be frustrating when you want to be out with friends who work normal nine-to-five jobs. It takes a lot of effort to organise nights out sometimes!' Working with sick children can be emotionally upsetting – so Emily says you need a positive attitude, bubbly personality and a good sense of humour to help you get through the bad days and to enjoy the good ones.

She offers the following advice to those wanting to work in the paediatric sector: 'Work with children before you apply to become a children's nurse; get lots of experience and make sure it's what you really want to do, because sick children can be very different in the way they act compared with well children.'

CHILD PROTECTION NURSING

The child protection nurse works with children on a one-to-one basis, as well as with their families, communities, self-help groups and pressure groups. Each strategic health authority in England and Wales has a designated nurse who works along with a designated doctor on child protection issues across all services. This involves teamwork with other agencies to help make sure all children are having their human rights respected. The designated nurse may be employed by a specific trust, but works across service boundaries. He/she acts as an important source of advice and represents the local health services on the area child protection committee.

CONSULTANT POSTS - NURSE, MIDWIFE AND HEALTH VISITOR

These newly created positions ensure that people using the NHS continue to benefit from the very best nursing and midwifery skills. The new nurse consultants spend a minimum of half their time working directly with patients, and are responsible for developing personal practice, being involved in research and evaluation, and contributing to education, training and development.

DAY SURGERY NURSING

Day surgery is for minor medical procedures where the patient can be discharged on the same day their surgery takes place. Day surgery nurses assess, plan, deliver and evaluate the care of their patients. Procedures can range from ear, nose and throat, oral, urology, plastic and cosmetic surgery to cataract removal, endoscopy, orthopaedic and pain-relief. Day surgery nurses manage patients' care from admission, assessment and preparation for surgery to monitoring and recovery after surgery and discharge management. Some units are attached to a theatre suite.

FANCY SOMETHING UNUSUAL?

Try nursing on holidays or expeditions! Expeditions are usually arduous and can involve many health hazards – from frostbite in the Arctic to sunstroke in the Sahara. The expedition nurse assists in the adequate preparation of expedition members, ensuring they have the best advice and information on health issues before departure. Then they monitor and help maintain the health and welfare of the expedition members whilst overseas. Expedition nurses must have a sound knowledge of first aid, and expedition organisations often look for nurses who have experience in A&E. Tropical disease experience or completion of a relevant course can also be useful. Contracts are usually for short periods only, varying from a couple of weeks to several months depending on the length of the expedition.

DERMATOLOGY NURSING

Our skin is our largest organ and there are many things that can go wrong with it. This means being a dermatology nurse is a very varied job. One day you could be treating acute cases of acne, the next patch-testing a patient with allergy problems. Dermatology nurses are often involved in clinical trials and audits and they may also use their expertise to teach patients to use camouflage make-up and wigs or to train other healthcare professionals. Many run their own clinics, where they carry out treatments such as the removal of warts, port wine stains and tattoos using ultraviolet light or laser procedures.

DISTRICT/COMMUNITY NURSING

District/community nurses are often based in GP surgeries. They work in partnership with patients and their carers in the community, assessing healthcare needs and developing appropriate packages of care.

FAMILY PLANNING NURSING

Family planning nurses provide contraceptive and sexual health advice as well as sexual health education. They also promote breast awareness and perform cervical smears. Many GP practice nurses fulfil the role of family planning nurse, but they also work in sexual health clinics, women's health centres, teenage clinics and abortion services.

FERTILITY NURSING

As more and more people, both couples and individuals, seek help in conceiving, the role of fertility nurse is becoming increasingly popular. They work in hospitals, in primary care, in the independent sector and in specialist fertility clinics or departments. They provide counselling, education and support to those undergoing fertility treatment and perform tests such as semen analysis, blood tests and imaging uterine cavities. They also perform procedures such as egg retrieval and sperm aspiration. Some fertility nurses run their own nurse-led clinics, which involves them in business planning and budget management.

GYNAECOLOGY NURSING

These days many women undergo some form of gynaecological treatment for conditions such as cysts, endometriosis and blocked fallopian tubes. Gynaecology nurses assess, plan and implement the care of these women before and after their gynaecological surgery. An important part of their role is to provide counselling and support to help alleviate patients' anxiety. They also give health advice. Some nurses run pre-admission clinics.

HAEMOPHILIA NURSING

Haemophilia is a serious genetic condition; haemophiliacs lack the clotting factor in blood, which means they bleed excessively with very slow clotting of the blood. Haemophilia nurses work in hospitals to plan, deliver and evaluate care given to any haemophiliac patients who are admitted. However, very few patients now require hospitalisation, so specialist nurses liaise between hospital and home, where patients and carers are taught how to administer treatment.

CASE STUDY – SENIOR STAFF NURSE, HAEMATOLOGY
Lucy Joyce is 28 years old. She first got interested in nursing at the age of 11, when she became a member of the St John Ambulance Brigade. She did A levels in home economics and human biology, and went on to do a diploma in adult nursing. She has recently completed a diploma in haematology nursing. Lucy works on the haematology ward at Leicester Royal Infirmary, Universities of Leicester NHS Trust.

'I am often in charge of a 22-bedded unit, where we treat many different abnormalities in the blood, some malignant and some not. Examples of these include sickle cell anaemia, leukaemia, lymphoma, thallasaemia, myloma and a huge variety of blood clotting disorders. I have to administer medication to the patients I have taken on that day, as well as giving IV (intravenous) drugs both to my patients and to those in other teams if their staff nurse is junior and has not been trained to administer them. This also includes giving patients multiple blood transfusions, which is a large part of the ward's workload. I am also trained to take any bloods the doctor may require.' She is also responsible for giving chemotherapy to patients on the ward and, if she is in charge of a shift, she will be responsible for bed management and finding new admissions a bed. Another aspect of her duties is to support junior staff and students.

Lucy loves her ward as the patients are often there for long periods and she gets to know them and their families. 'I am

---

able to support them through a time that is often difficult and give them a high level of care, whatever the outcome,' she says. 'I love the fact that I can teach others the skills that I have learnt and help them become better nurses. My ward has a mixture of very ill patients and others who need very little support. I also like the variety in my job as I feel that no day is ever the same and there is little opportunity to get bored.'

Lucy views nursing as a continual learning process as you progress in your role, and she is very prepared to go on different courses in order to further that progression. In fact, Lucy is now going to start a degree in nursing and aims to become a deputy sister.

However, she does find it difficult when she and the rest of the team are unable to successfully treat patients or control their condition. The success rate for treating malignant haematology conditions is less than 50% so deaths are quite common. She believes you have to be quite tough as a nurse as you can have bad days – for example, where your favourite patient dies – yet you still have to go back to work the next day.

You also need to be very committed as most nursing posts work on a shift system which means your social life may suffer. Because of this, she says: 'Think about it very carefully, as you have to be very committed to do this job, sometimes with very little reward. If possible, try and get some experience before you start your training as this will help you see what the job entails and also give you some basic experience. I worked as a healthcare assistant before I started my nurse training and this helped me decide whether it was the correct career choice.'

HEALTH VISITOR

All health visitors are qualified nurses who have taken a further degree programme to qualify as a health visitor. They enter a family's life in the first weeks after a child's birth and carry out developmental screening. They also provide health education programmes for individuals and communities. Some health visitors are attached to doctors' surgeries, while others visit people in their homes and schools within their own specific area. They work in conjunction with a network of other groups concerned with health, sickness, social and educational services. Once again, their work is very varied so they could be counselling the previous partners of someone diagnosed HIV positive, paying visits to mothers who have postnatal depression or supporting and advising someone who wants to give up smoking.

IN-FLIGHT NURSING

If you are taken ill on holiday it is the in-flight nurse who will escort you on the plane back to your own country. The flight may take place on a scheduled plane or on a dedicated aircraft or air ambulance. They not only provide care while on board the plane, but also on the journeys from or to the hospital and back to the patient's home. They make the initial health assessment and ensure both the patient's property and any medical equipment they are using is safely transferred along with the patient.

WORKING WITH THE PHARMACEUTICAL INDUSTRY
Ashfield Healthcare is a major provider of contract resources to the UK and Irish pharmaceutical industries. Part of the United Drug Group, it offers a range of services including sales force resourcing, nurse advisors, vacancy management and training and development.

All nurse advisors are qualified, registered nurses, protected by and working within the guidelines of the NMC Code of Conduct and the Association of the British Pharmaceutical Industry (ABPI) Code of Practice. The role provides an opportunity to specialise in one or two particular disease areas, with increasing emphasis on promoting health improvements and helping to fulfil demanding clinical targets. Raising the standards in particular disease areas can be of huge benefit to all parties involved with a Nurse Advisor Project, which makes the role such a fulfilling one. Firstly, the surgery benefits as they are concentrating on raising the standard of care and meeting clinical targets. More importantly, the patient benefits from the outcome and maybe a drug/therapy change, and the sponsoring pharmaceutical company gains recognition for sponsoring this additional expert resource that has helped to raise the standards of care. The nurse is in contact with many different GP practices, all with different ways of thinking, different policies and different ideas, yet all sharing the same priority of a high standard of patient care.

There are many different objectives for each project, which can include:

- Data trawling

- Auditing and producing detailed reports for individual surgeries

- Reviewing patient therapy and recommending changes to drugs/dosages

- Administering to patients

- Educating both patients and health professionals within the disease therapy area

- Raising the profile of the sponsoring company.

Work is carried out on a local, regional and sometimes national level, in conjunction with primary healthcare teams, pharmaceutical advisors, primary care teams and other health professionals. The work of a nurse advisor varies from day to day, week to week. The nurse advisor is responsible for filling their own diary and building up a manageable workload. This requires self-motivation and flexibility, and the results to be gained are both satisfying and rewarding.

(Source: Ashfield Healthcare – www.ashfieldhealthcare.com; used with permission)

LEARNING DISABILITY NURSING

Nationally, 3% of the population has a learning disability and nurses who qualify in this branch help them to live independent and fulfilling lives. Many learning disability nurses work with people in supported accommodation where three or four people with learning disabilities live together in flats or houses, with 24-hour support. Others work with individuals who require more intensive support in hospitals, or in specialist secure units for offenders with learning disabilities. Learning disability nurses may specialise in areas such as epilepsy, or working with people with sensory impairment.

LIAISON AND DISCHARGE PLANNING NURSING

Liaison and discharge planning nurses work in hospitals to develop effective policy and practice for the discharge of patients when they are ready to go home. This involves close liaison with primary care teams, other specialist agencies and bed management services.

MACMILLAN NURSING

Macmillan Cancer Support improves the lives of people affected by cancer – providing practical, medical, emotional and financial support and pushing for better cancer care. Macmillan nurses provide expert information, advice and support both to people with cancer and to their families. They also support and advise other healthcare professionals. They are Registered Nurses with at least five years' experience, including two or more years in cancer or palliative care.

Macmillan nurses are usually employed by the NHS – Macmillan Cancer Support sets up their position, and pays for it for a set time – usually the first three years. Then the NHS (or other partner organisation) takes on responsibility for managing and paying them, but Macmillan continues to educate and support them.

There are around 2900 Macmillan nurses throughout the UK. They include community care and hospital support nurses, and others who specialise in particular cancers, treatments or other specialist areas of cancer care; for example Macmillan breast care nurses, Macmillan paediatric nurses, or Macmillan chemotherapy nurses. Macmillan lead cancer nurses are senior nurse managers who help shape the future of cancer and palliative care services in their area.

More information is available from www.macmillan.org.uk.
(Source: Courtesy of Macmillan Cancer Support)

MENTAL HEALTH NURSING

Mental health nurses work with GPs, psychiatrists, social workers and others to coordinate the care of people suffering from mental illness. They form therapeutic relationships with mentally ill people (and their families), helping them to maintain independence, to manage their condition and to overcome the stigma attached to mental illness. Part of the training for mental health nurses involves learning to control challenging behaviour and defuse tense or violent situations.

Mental health nurses may also work in forensic settings providing care and treatment for mentally disordered offenders. **Forensic mental health nurses** will have a caseload of patients for whom they assess and implement nursing care in medium- or high-security establishments and also in the community. If they work within a ward they are responsible for risk assessment and risk management procedures and must integrate security protocols with nursing practise. They supervise the practise of nursing students and other, unregistered nursing staff, and provide effective clinical leadership within their team. They must also maintain quality standards and undertake health promotion activities.

MULTIPLE SCLEROSIS SPECIALIST NURSING

The Multiple Sclerosis (MS) specialist is a relatively new role in nursing. They have extensive caseloads of clients with multiple sclerosis and use their specialised expertise on those who are just undergoing diagnostic investigation as well as those who have already been diagnosed and have severe disability. They liaise with social and community services, primary care teams (including GPs) and hospitals. You must be a skilled communicator and educator in order to undertake this role.

NATIONAL BLOOD SERVICE

There are a variety of career opportunities in the National Blood Service due to the ongoing demand for blood, increasing commitments in tissue banking and the changing needs of the NHS. For more information, see www.blood.co.uk, or contact the National Nurse Advisor, National Blood Service, Oak House, Reeds Crescent, Watford, Hertfordshire WD1 1QH or call 01923 486800.

NURSE EDUCATIONALIST

Nurse educationalists work in the practice setting, delivering both higher education and further education. Nurse lecturers teach and assess in higher education establishments and are responsible for pre- and post-registration nursing or midwifery curriculum design. They also undertake research projects and provide pastoral care and individual tutorial support for students. Practice educators work in a practice setting and are responsible for teaching and development. Further education lecturers work mainly with post-16 year olds and/or adult learners. Nurses find employment in the further education sector through teaching on health and social care-related courses including Access to Nursing/Healthcare and NVQ/SVQ programmes.

NURSERY NURSE AND PLAY SPECIALIST

Nursery nurses work with children aged from 0 to 7 years in a variety of settings which might include local authority or privately owned nurseries or nursery, infant and specialist schools. Some specialise so they can work with children who are physically disabled or have learning difficulties or mental health problems.

Nursery nurses are responsible for the social and educational development as well as the physical well-being of their young charges. They plan and supervise activities including reading, arts and crafts, music and cooking and monitor and observe their children, sometimes making reports on a child's development. They will work closely with parents and report any concerns. They are also responsible for feeding, changing and bathing the children in their care.

Further information is available from the Council for Awards in Children's Care and Education (CACHE) – see www.cache.org.uk or call 01727 818616.

Hospital play specialists help children express their feelings through play. They plan and supervise activities with children in hospital so that play can be used as a means of communication, educating them about their illnesses and allying any misplaced worries they may have in order to reduce anxiety. They encourage children to develop their creative skills to show their thoughts and worries relating to hospital, helping them to adapt to any restrictions they may have resulting from hospitalisation.

Further information is available from the National Association of Hospital Play Staff (NAHPS) – see www.nahps.org.uk.

CASE STUDY – CRECHE MANAGER
When 35-year-old Sue Modeva left school she went to Southport College to do her Nursery Nurse training via the Nursery Nurses Education Board (NNEB). However, she left after a year and did not take up childcare again until after her

son was old enough to go to primary school. She then started to work in the nursery at his school and was later offered a position to assist with children with special needs. She was working part-time and earning, but she also started to train on the job to become a Specialist Teacher's Assistant. A high percentage of the children she worked with not only had special needs but also had English as a second language. Her duties included building relationships with the children and implementing play strategies. Five years ago she became the crèche manager at a Cannons gym in London and she updated her qualifications by attending a part-time evening course for two years giving her a Cache level 3 Certificate of Professional Development in Work with Children and Young People.

'Here I am still very hands on with the children, but I now have to deal with legal requirements, monitoring my staff, recruiting, doing performance evaluations and liasing with outside agencies such as Child Protection,' she says. Five hundred children between the ages of three months and five years are registered at her crèche and they probably get between 44 and 50 children a day as their mums come into the gym. For Sue, the interaction with the children is the highlight of the day and she says it keeps her young, although she emphasises the work can be extremely tiring both emotionally and physically, especially as having eye contact with the children requires a lot of bending down and a lot of picking up. She believes in order to make a success of working in a crèche or nursery you need the following strengths: 'You really need to be patient to do this job and have self-confidence and be committed and caring. Above all you have to have the right attitude and be responsible and reliable. Liking babies is not enough because in this job you have to constantly develop and update your skills in line with new legislation.'

If you are interested in becoming a nursery nurse Sue suggests contacting your local Early Years Development Partnership (EYDP) who will have a list of nurseries who may be willing to give you work experience, or get involved with your local Brownies, Cubs or Rainbow group. She also suggests babysitting and joining a drama group as role-play and reading stories are key areas in childcare. As far as progression through the industry is concerned you can always move up by becoming a manager but also think about branching out into child psychology, or into education through drama. Ultimately, Sue would like to have her own small nursery.

NURSING ASSISTANT/HEALTHCARE ASSISTANT

You don't actually need any specific qualifications to become a nursing assistant or a healthcare assistant in a hospital, you just need to be enthusiastic about caring for people. However, within 12 months of employment you must undertake training to gain the National Vocational Qualification level 2 in Care. Most nursing assistants work shifts and their duties include taking patients' temperatures and pulses and recording them, helping nursing staff to move patients, and assisting patients with washing, eating and drinking. They work in many areas within the hospital including outpatient clinics, maternity, elderly care and even operating theatres. For a more detailed look at the care professions, see *Real Life Guides: Care* (Trotman Publishing, 2006).

CASE STUDY – NURSING ASSISTANT/STUDENT NURSE
Maxine Holder-Critchlow started her career as a qualified nursery nurse and went on to work for a series of nurseries while being employed by an agency. It was the agency that asked Maxine to go and work at famous children's hospital Great Ormond Street (GOS) in order to help out the nurses who had a very heavy workload. She started out entertaining the children, taking them down to the x-ray department or to have scans, and bottle or tube feeding the babies.

Her manager decided it would be better if she worked with the long-term patients and she became an associate carer or nursing assistant, learning to care for patients with tracheotomies and even accompanying them on visits home. The longer she stayed, the more experienced she became – and when she reached the point where she was on the highest level of pay for an associate carer she decided to train to be a nurse. She has just started her training at London South Bank University and in three years she will qualify as a Registered Children's Nurse (RCN).

Maxine says: 'The best part of my job is if you have been nursing a child who has been really poorly and they come back to the ward and ask to see you, and you realise the difference in them – just how well they have become; that's what makes the job worthwhile. I'm getting to do the thing I love the most and that is working with children.'

Although she is enjoying her training, she says she does miss being at the hospital and is really looking forward to her forthcoming six-week block release placement at GOS. 'It's really interesting because before, I only had the practical experience; now, with what I am learning, it is all making sense to me – now I know why I do what I do.'

In five years' time Maxine would like to be an S Grade nurse, which is a Senior Staff Nurse, because then she would have the opportunity to actually take charge of a ward and she wants to further her career by doing more training in order to keep up with new procedures.

Her advice to anyone wanting to become a nursing assistant is: 'First and foremost you have to want to do it – your heart must be in it because the biggest downside of this business is if one of your patients doesn't make it and that is the hardest, hardest thing; some people can't take that. You need to be very kind, very patient with people, and you have to be very understanding and have good listening skills. Nursing is hard work and you are on your feet a lot, but you get so focused on what you are doing you look at the clock and think "where has the time gone?"'

The post has been set up to respond to the increasing numbers of clergy who are suffering with stress, leading to some being off work for long periods, and a few taking early retirement on health grounds. The coordinator will be 48-year-old mother of two Julie Barrett, who has been working near Bristol as a psychotherapist in private practice.

While working as a nurse, Julie developed her counselling skills, and then spent some time managing support services in mental health housing before going freelance. She is an active member of the Church of England, has been licensed as a Reader (authorised lay minister) since 2001, and is a member of the Franciscan Third Order. Julie also assists in the chaplaincy of a prison.

PAIN MANAGEMENT SPECIALIST NURSING

Palliative care professionals usually deal with pain caused by malignancy (cancer) while nurses who specialise in pain management work in both acute and chronic pain teams. In acute pain management, nurses play a vital role in ensuring the safe and effective treatment of pain caused by surgery, trauma or disease. They educate nurses and other healthcare professionals about new pain-relieving techniques, audit treatment options and may undertake research. They work with medical staff, physiotherapists, pharmacists, psychologists and occupational therapists to devise pain management programmes for their patients, who usually attend a structured programme on a group basis once or twice a week. Nurses play a role in monitoring the patient's use of medication and help them to plan a drug reduction programme if so wished.

PRACTICE NURSING

You've probably already come across a practice nurse as a patient when you were a child – he/she would have given you your jabs and boosters! They work alongside the doctors in general practice surgeries and health centres and they perform a range of tasks, freeing up the doctors' precious time. They manage health promotion clinics including travel health (advising which jabs you need in order to visit certain countries), immunisations and sexual and reproductive health (performing women's regular cervical smears), breast awareness and even 'stop smoking' counselling. They are involved in the recognition of conditions such as diabetes and asthma.

PRISON NURSING

Inmates must have proper access to healthcare and this is provided by prison doctors and nurses. Nurses make health assessments on inmates by observation and screening, and help prisoners to manage conditions such as diabetes, epilepsy, asthma, and drug and alcohol dependence. A large part of the job is to promote health via exercise, diet and adopting a healthier lifestyle (by giving up smoking/drugs). Prison nurses also care for inmates with mental health problems and often work with community psychiatric nurses to provide support for those at risk of self-harm, bullying, suicide or depression.

REHABILITATION NURSING

Rehabilitation nurses work in specialist hospital or community rehabilitation units, day care units, nurse-led clinics, continuing care and intermediate care. Some nurses work with specific clients, such as those with spinal injuries, stroke victims, those with cardiac disease or older people. They assess each individual client's needs before drawing up rehabilitation plans for them and take a leading role in coordinating treatment with the other carers, family members and healthcare workers involved in each case. They also educate those involved about the rehabilitation process and act as counsellors to their clients.

DOING SOMETHING DIFFERENT – NURSING OPPORTUNITIES IN NEW ZEALAND

If you fancy working abroad as a nurse, one attractive option is to work in New Zealand. Nursing work in New Zealand is similar to that in the UK. The hospitals are run by District Health Boards (DHBs), and conditions within these hospitals are good, with many having recently been upgraded. The hospitals vary in size from small 150-bed rural hospitals to 500-bed tertiary care facilities.

Most nurses work eight-hour shifts that include night duty. Many hospitals have, or are introducing, 'clinical career pathways' – nurses working on a career pathway are paid according to the level they have achieved. Other nurses are paid according to their years of experience.

In order to be eligible to work in New Zealand you need to apply for a Working Holiday Visa or Work Permit in the UK from the New Zealand High Commission. Although it is not compulsory to join the New Zealand Nursing Organisation (the national union for nursing and midwifery staff) it is advisable as you will then be covered by the Nursing Unions & Indemnity Insurance.

RESEARCH NURSING

Research nurses can work in various areas including universities (where many hold a combined teaching role), in clinical settings and in the pharmaceutical industry. Depending on their level of seniority they identify and screen suitable patients for trials (where relevant) and get their informed consent, develop and design research protocols, coordinate and undertake data collection from the trials, and supply patient support. They write reports and analyse data and disseminate their findings; some even publish papers. Many will be involved with submitting proposals and finding funding for research projects.

RESUSCITATION OFFICER

Resuscitation officers are responsible for the planning, organisation and implementation of resuscitation training for healthcare professionals.

RHEUMATOLOGY NURSING

There are over 20 million people in the UK suffering from rheumatic conditions such as rheumatoid arthritis and metabolic bone diseases such as osteoporosis. Specialist rheumatology nurses work in the community, hospital wards, outpatient clinics, research and education. They assist patients and their carers in coming to terms with the physical, psychological and social effects of their disease and they help their patients to manage their pain. They may run nurse-led clinics and give advice on treatment options. They work closely with other healthcare professionals such as GPs and physiotherapists in order to obtain the very best course of care for their patients.

SCHOOL NURSING

School nurses are employed either by a Primary Care Trust, NHS Trust in Wales, Health Board in Scotland, Health and Social Services Board in Northern Ireland or directly by the school, if it is independent. They undertake health interviews, administer immunisation programmes, carry out developmental screening and provide health and sex education within the school environment.

SEXUAL HEALTH NURSING

Sexual health includes testing for and treating HIV, family planning and sexually transmitted disease services. Some clinics specialise in offering support and advice to young people. Work in this area is very varied and includes pre- and post-test counselling, actually carrying out the diagnostic tests and health assessments, and providing advice on treatment. Those working with young people may well be involved in outreach projects in schools, hostels and colleges.

TELEPHONE ADVICE AND CONSULTATION

As people's lives get more hectic and their time more stretched, it's no wonder the opportunities for nurses to provide information, advice and guidance over the telephone have grown so rapidly. NHS Direct is the largest telephone health advice and consultation service in the world and operates in England and Wales (and Scotland has recently set up NHS 24).

NHS Direct provides the public with the opportunity to obtain advice on health matters from qualified nurses over the phone – so no more sitting around crowded GP waiting rooms for common complaints such as colds. NHS Direct sites also employ health information advisors, who give information about local health and social services, self-help groups, charities and common health conditions. Four or five years' post-registration experience is usually needed to become an NHS Direct nurse advisor.

THEATRE NURSING (PERIOPERATIVE NURSING)

Theatre nurses are responsible for the care and safety of patients undergoing surgical procedures. As is to be expected in such a complicated field there are many specialised nursing posts available, including:

- **Anaesthetic nurses** care for the patient before, during and after the induction of anaesthesia. They also ensure relevant equipment and medication is prepared and ready for use

- **Scrub nurses** assist the surgeon(s) during the surgical procedure by preparing instruments and assisting in their use. They pass correct instruments to the surgeon and ensure nothing is left inside the patient during or after the operation

- **Circulating nurses** are responsible for the environment outside the sterile field and assist in creating and maintaining a safe surgical environment

- **Recovery room nurses** care for and monitor the patient recovering from the immediate effects of surgery and anaesthesia. This includes monitoring vital signs, urine output, wound dressings and maintaining intravenous fluids. Communication between recovery room nurses and critical care staff is essential to ensure appropriate continuing care for the patient when they leave surgery

- **First assistants** use their specialist knowledge and skills to carry out risk management, infection control, wound management and suturing of wounds.

TROPICAL DISEASES

Following training in nursing, you might choose to specialise in tropical diseases. In this area you would deal with travellers on both a long-term and short-term basis suffering from such conditions as leprosy and malaria that they have contracted overseas. Nurses screen and test for parasites and viruses and are responsible for administering drugs and the overall well-being of patients. For queries relating to further training in the field of tropical disease, contact the Hospital for Tropical Diseases (www.thehtd.org) or Liverpool School of Tropical Medicine (www.liv.ac.uk/lstm). The London School of Hygiene and Tropical Medicine runs a Tropical Nursing Course – for more information visit www.lshtm.ac.uk. (There is also more information on the content of this course in Chapter 5.)

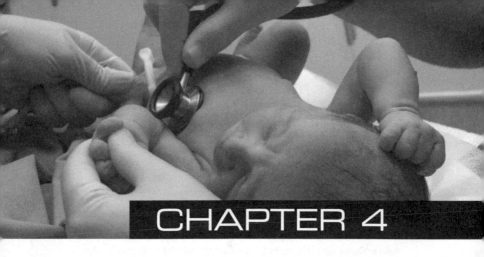

CHAPTER 4

Where midwifery could take you

WHAT'S MIDWIFERY ALL ABOUT?

You may think that being a midwife is all about working with babies – but in fact this is a misconception: midwifery is really all about working with women. This chapter looks in more detail at the role of midwife and at what the job is like, before exploring some of the different job specialisations on offer.

WHAT DO MIDWIVES DO?

Midwives support and care for women throughout pregnancy, labour, delivery and into the first phase of postnatal care. They also support and care for the partners and families of pregnant women and new mothers, as this can be a highly stressful time for everyone. They help new parents to adapt to their new roles and provide education and support on such subjects as bathing and breastfeeding.

Midwives are highly trained, multi-skilled healthcare professionals. Though they work as part of a multi-disciplinary team, liaising and working in partnership with other healthcare professionals, they enjoy a high level of responsibility and independence. A woman can expect to have all her antenatal (before the baby is born) and postnatal (after the baby is born) care needs met by midwives and it is only in the most serious cases, where problems arise, that this is not the case.

FASCINATING FACTS

In 2001 at Rosie Hospital (the maternity unit for Addenbrooke's Hospital, part of Cambridge University Hospitals Trust), 4500 babies were delivered. Midwives were present at 100% of the births and were actually responsible for 59.6% of those deliveries.

(Source: Addenbrooke's Hospital)

Because the midwife is present at every birth, whether at home or in hospital, she touches everyone's life. She is usually the first and main contact for the expectant mother during her pregnancy, and throughout labour and the postnatal period. A large part of what she does is to offer emotional support – midwives do not make decisions for women but they are there to provide the right support and information so that women can make their own informed choices about the care they receive before, during and after pregnancy. The midwife informs the mothers about the services and options available, such as writing a Birthing Plan which sets out what pain relief (if any) she wishes to have during labour, and whether she would like the use of a birthing pool. Midwives also perform any antenatal screening and diagnostic procedures their patients may need and will support them for up to 28 days after the birth – although if the mum and baby are fine this period usually shrinks to around 10 or 11 days.

Every delivery is a major event in the lives of the people involved. Midwives have the lead professional role in preparing for and managing the event, intervening where necessary and knowing what to do if the mother or baby is sick. Women from all walks of life, cultural backgrounds and (increasingly) from all age groups have babies, so midwives provide professional support and reassurance to a huge diversity of women, during a very intense and emotional experience. That's why they have to stay calm and alert in times of stress, and enable women to feel confident and in control. On the rare occasions when something goes wrong, they have to be ready to react quickly and effectively.

WHAT ARE THE WORKING CONDITIONS?

Midwives work shift patterns to provide continual support for women day and night. They are responsible for their own individual practice and have a statutory responsibility to keep up to date with current knowledge. All midwives (including those in the independent sector) must have a named 'supervisor of midwives' to assist them with updating their knowledge and to ensure their practice is safe. It is the only profession that has supervision to protect the public from incompetent practitioners.

The vast majority of midwives work for the NHS in maternity units, attached to GP surgeries, in health centres and also in patients' homes. However, there are also independent (self-employed) midwives in the UK – mostly assisting women with home births – and midwives working in private-sector hospitals.

FASCINATING FACTS

Midwives working in NHS maternity units spend roughly 75% of their time in hospitals and 25% out in the community.

As mentioned in Chapter 1, the new NHS pay system Agenda for Change (AfC) is in the process of being introduced throughout the UK. Entry level for midwives is normally Band 5 (£17,660), but midwife consultants can earn up to £48,185. There are also special allowances (for being on-call or working over weekends or on public holidays) and weightings for living in and around London that can further boost your earnings – see Chapter 1 for further details. Independent midwives usually work at around Grade G level, which is likely to mean a salary of between £25,245 and £30,720, depending on seniority.

CASE STUDY – MIDWIFE SUPERVISOR
It was after she had her first child that 35-year-old Laura Abbot decided to do her midwifery training. She trained as a nurse at St Batholomew's in London and, having gained her RGN and Diploma in nursing, went to work in intensive care and gained a specialist ITU qualification and a degree in Healthcare. After five years as a nurse she trained as a midwife at the University of Hertfordshire and gained her RM qualification as well as a BSc(Hons).

She then worked within the NHS in a busy birth centre and delivery suite but decided to leave to become a self-employed independent midwife, supporting women who choose to give birth at home. Recently, she was nominated to take a supervisors of midwives preparation course and is now an appointed supervisor of midwives for the eastern region of England. She is now taking a Master's degree.

Laura has a caseload of women who book her to support them throughout their pregnancies, during the birth and for around six weeks after the baby has been born. She says 'I have a close relationship with the families I work with, visiting them in their own homes – by the time the baby is ready to be born we all know each other very well and have a trusting relationship, which is very important when the labour starts!'

She cares for the women physically, undertaking checks during pregnancy – including checking for the size and position of the baby and looking for any signs of illnesses such as pre-eclampsia. 'For most women, pregnancy is a time of health – so I look at things to enhance health such as optimum nutrition,' she says. However, most of what Laura does involves getting to know each woman emotionally and helping her work through any past issues, such as previous traumatic births. She stays with her clients throughout the labour and birth and helps them with issues such as breastfeeding after the birth, giving lots of emotional support. 'Sometimes, just having someone at the end of the phone is a great support to women,' she explains. She tailors her care to each individual woman but usually visits every few weeks until the later stages of pregnancy and then daily for the first week postnatally.

She loves being in such a privileged position, at such an amazing and special time in someone's life, and is very much enjoying the challenge of being a supervisor of midwives, which gives her the dual role of protecting the public and supporting midwives. 'I would like to work with more midwives, both inside and outside the NHS,' she says. She loves teaching and she regularly talks at the University of Hertfordshire on subjects such as normality of childbirth, homebirth and waterbirth. She says the downside of what she does is the fact it can be very emotionally draining and she has to be careful to take holidays to recharge her batteries.

If you want to be a successful midwife, Laura advises that you must be: 'approachable, hard-working, self-aware, friendly and professional and, most of all, woman-centred.' You need to research your local maternity services and to speak to pregnant women in order to find out what they say they need from their midwives. 'Midwifery is not all about lovely babies – you also need to look at issues such as poverty and vulnerable women, child protection and domestic violence. Finally, explore how you feel about women's issues, inequalities, breastfeeding, birth and pregnancy.'

WHAT MAKES A GOOD MIDWIFE?

There are a number of skills and personal qualities that could make you ideally suited to being a midwife. These include:

- A real love of working with women and acting in their best interests

- The ability to get on with individuals from all backgrounds – you need to be a 'people' person

- Communication skills and the ability to work in a team

- The ability to take responsibility and work on your own initiative

- A calm, controlled disposition – and the ability to retain this, even in high-pressure situations where you need to be able to think on your feet

- Good organisational skills and the ability and inclination to keep accurate records and write accurate reports

- Flexibility and adaptability – sometimes babies arrive when you least expect them, so be prepared to drop everything at a minute's notice!

Have a think about the points mentioned above and try to work out whether you've got what it takes. If you think you have, read on – the next section looks at the different jobs available and uses case studies to give you a taste of what the work is really like.

WHAT MIDWIFERY JOBS ARE OUT THERE?

MATERNITY CARE ASSISTANT

Maternity care assistants help the midwives in their duties by restocking clinical areas, keeping the ward tidy and (most importantly) clean, transporting specimens to pathology, assisting pregnant women in going to the bathroom, bathing and taking refreshments, assisting with teaching baby care, clearing up after a delivery, and taking and recording temperature and blood pressure.

You don't need formal qualifications to become a maternity care assistant. However, you do need to complete a probationary period as a nursing assistant before undertaking specialised NVQ level 1 training.

CASE STUDY – PART-TIME MIDWIFE

Forty-five-year-old mother of four Fiona Davis originally trained as a nurse at Carshalton Beeches in Surrey and from there decided to train as a health visitor. At the time (the 1980s), in order to become a health visitor, you had to complete part of your midwifery training – so she applied to Epsom, where she did an additional 18-month midwifery course. It soon became clear to her that it was midwifery that she wanted to concentrate on and she started work in that capacity in the Chobham and Oxshot areas. While there, her unit won a global award for being Baby Friendly and promoting breastfeeding, and this is the area she has been involved in ever since.

She took her Teaching and Assessing in Midwifery ENB (English National Board) 997/998 in 1992, and in August 2005 she started working part-time at St George's Hospital in Tooting, London. Here, she does two six-hour days a week on the postnatal ward, specifically concentrating on mums and breastfeeding and any problems they may have. Her allocation for a shift is between six to eight mums and their babies.

'I like supporting women with the decisions they have made, making motherhood an enjoyable experience. Working on the postnatal ward I don't get to see the women for very long so it is about making them see and understand (about breastfeeding). The delight for me is having someone who goes off and I know is going to continue to breastfeed and is going to enjoy it, rather than going home with sore nipples and giving up at the first opportunity.'

The downside for Fiona is the time constraints that occur because of a lack of staff and the sheer workload this causes. Although St George's has a commitment to be Baby Friendly, Fiona sometimes feels new mums do not get the total support they need because there are just not enough staff to supply it.

> She says you need adaptability and a caring approach to do what she does. 'You should never do midwifery just because you think it's a good degree to do – you have to have some form of vocation to make a success of it. You really have to be someone who likes working with people and it is very much about being with the woman so you need to have an understanding of women. I'd say go out and get some real life experiences before deciding to do this; do some voluntary work and get some experience working with children either in a hospital environment or within the community, because that will really hone your people skills.'

COMMUNITY MIDWIFERY

Community midwives first see women after about ten weeks of pregnancy and continue to provide care either in the doctor's surgery or at the woman's home. During the antenatal period, they offer:

- Screening

- Full antenatal surveillance

- Parent education

- Advice on all issues relating to pregnancy

- Information on choices for labour and delivery

- Discussion regarding infant feeding.

After the birth, community midwives provide care and support in the parents' home.

CASE STUDY - FULL-TIME MIDWIFE

Although she originally trained as an actress, 47-year-old Terie Seignior decided to retrain as a midwife once she had her second child. Firstly, she became involved with the National Childbirth Trust, through which she did a certificate to teach antenatal classes. This enabled her to keep up to date with maternity issues. Then, after the birth of her third child, she did a BSc degree in Midwifery at King's College, London. She qualified in 2002 and since then has been working on the labour ward at King's. She also spent a year with a community midwifery group practice specialising in pregnant women with diabetes and with HIV. She now works as a Band 7 midwife, coordinating the labour ward and mentoring student midwives.

Terie works 12-hour shifts; a day shift starts at 7.15am and a night shift starts at 7.15pm. At the beginning of each shift she receives the handover from the previous coordinator and then allocates the new midwives on duty to various cases depending on what is required. She accompanies the doctors on their ward rounds and tries to keep things as normal as possible. 'All the time there are different women coming in for a variety of reasons – from experiencing pains to being in labour – and it's my job to prioritise each need and then allocate them a room and a midwife to care for them; not all that easy given our workload of almost 5000 births last year! I am also responsible for making sure each midwife, healthcare assistant and our receptionist gets their break,' she explains.

'It has been a fantastic few years and I really love my job,' she says. 'It's a real privilege to be present at the start of life, and to enable it to happen as naturally as possible is a great bonus!' She says she loves every aspect of her job: 'It's great enabling normal labour, water births, and breech births to happen,' she says. 'It's also rewarding to encourage doctors to see normal labour and births and be able to give care when things don't go as planned, and to be empathetic and respectful. I also enjoy challenging the doctors and making sure their solution really is a solution and not just a pathway to the theatre!'

Terie would love to get involved with research that promotes midwifery-led care and says that if you want to do what she does, you need to be a good listener, empathetic, an advocate, a supporter and someone who can solve problems easily. Most of all, she says you should just do it. 'It's an amazingly challenging and rewarding job where no two days are the same. You get to meet so many interesting people and it's a continual learning environment!'

INDEPENDENT MIDWIFE

Independent midwives (IMs) are fully qualified midwives who have chosen to work outside the NHS in a self-employed capacity. The role encompasses the care of women during pregnancy, birth and afterwards. IMs offer continuity of care, and empower women to make informed choices and decisions at every stage.

The services of IMs are most often requested for home births, and the rest are for planned hospital births. They accompany their clients into all hospitals, their roles depending on local arrangements and clients' needs. However, an IM cannot act as the midwife in the hospital unless she has a contract with the local Trust. She must otherwise act as birth partner, with the hospital's own midwife taking over during labour. IMs liaise with other healthcare practitioners if and when necessary and can arrange all screenings and diagnostic tests, such as scans and blood tests, either through the NHS or privately. Should the desired place of birth or type of care need to change at any time, IMs can assist clients in achieving this as smoothly and gently as possible. IMs always see the care of their clients through to 28 days after the birth.

CASE STUDY – INDEPENDENT MIDWIFE
Having done a sociology degree, 51-year-old Annie Francis originally trained to be a social worker, but it was the experiences of having her own four children that convinced

her that her vocation was elsewhere. Having been labelled high risk with her first, breech birth, which she had in hospital, for her second baby Annie employed an independent midwife and opted to have the baby at home – this was such a happy experience her mind was made up and she went on to do a direct entry three-year full-time diploma in midwifery. She qualified in September 1998 and went to work at King's Hospital, part of the NHS, in October of the same year. Within four months she knew that working for the NHS was not for her and she switched to the independent sector. She now works in a self-employed capacity for the South London Independent Midwives practice with two colleagues.

Women find us through the internet or through the Independent Midwives Association (IMA), but mainly through word of mouth. We each have primary clients but we work as a pair so every woman has a second midwife. We mostly work with women who want home births because we can't be midwives in NHS or private hospitals because of contracts, insurance and protocols – we can only be birth partners in a hospital.

'When a woman takes us on, we visit throughout the pregnancy and do all the things NHS midwives do – we listen to the baby, check its growth, check the mother's well-being and, most importantly, we explore the journey the mother wants to take. Maybe they have had a bad experience before or have issues we will discuss and explore. We are available 24 hours a day, seven days a week, so we are always on-call and that can be challenging, so you really have to think about that if you want to be an independent midwife.

'I'm passionate about home births because I believe it is a much safer way for women to birth their babies unless there are risk factors. My colleagues and I are advocates of women having genuine choice. Our clients often cope brilliantly through labour because they know what to expect and what is happening and they are well supported.'

In fact, many of Annie's clients cope so well they don't even need pain relief, although she has gas and air, Tens

(Transcutaneous Electrical Nerve Stimulator) and birthing pools available for them. Annie will also stay with her clients for between six and eight weeks after the birth, offering advice on breastfeeding and keeping an eye on both mother and baby.

'I love the fact that I am doing something that doesn't feel like a job. I love every moment of it, even when it is hard. It's the most extraordinary job and it has huge rewards. I embrace it all – I'm not just working on a labour ward, I'm doing all of it all of the time and I love the variety. Yes, there are downsides, such as the times when babies do not survive. That is very, very hard. It is completely devastating and this is why every midwife has a supervisory midwife to talk her through things like that.'

According to Annie, some members of the medical profession see independent midwives as mavericks, and this can lead them to feel rather exposed. Also, she points out that there is no insurance available for independent midwives, so if someone decides to sue, the individual midwife gets sued personally.

Annie lists the strengths you must have to succeed as an independent midwife as: 'Thinking on your feet; and everything you do must be done with integrity. You have to be very honest and be able to cope with traumas and you must have some life skills so go out and do some living. Finally, ask yourself why you want to do this – don't do it if you are thinking of working with children because that is just a tiny bit of it. You have to love being with women. It isn't glamorous but it is wonderfully rewarding.'

PROMOTION

There are good promotion prospects within midwifery, with a lot of different roles open to qualified midwives. For example, midwives with experience can:

- Take on increased responsibility as a supervisor or manager of a ward or unit

- Become a clinical specialist

- Become a consultant midwife

- Research and develop special areas of practice, such as public health or women's health

- Become involved in or run specialist services such as family planning and teenage pregnancy clinics

- Work abroad

- Move sideways into research or education.

Here are a few of the job roles you might find open up to you:

- **Practice development/research midwife**: in this role, the midwife leads projects designed to improve care by working with colleagues in the clinical setting

- **Midwifery risk manager**: it's a sad fact of life that sometimes things do go wrong and the risk manager is there to review such incidents and to suggest changes to policy if need be

- **Ultrasound midwife**: the use of ultrasound to monitor the foetus's development and growth is now commonplace and ultrasound midwives are trained to recognise exactly what it is they are seeing on the monitor and to pick up on any anomalies or irregularities

- **NVQ coordinator**: this qualified member of staff is involved in the training of more junior staff, for example in helping nursing assistants become maternity care assistants by successfully completing NVQ level 2. NVQ coordinators develop training programmes, assessments and examinations.

A FEW KEY ORGANISATIONS
The Royal College of Midwives (RCM)
The RCM is the oldest and largest professional midwifery organisation in the world. Founded in 1881, it has more than 38,000 members and represents more than 95% of working midwives in the UK. It is the only trade union and professional organisation run by midwives for midwives. It is the voice of midwifery, providing excellence in professional leadership, education, influence and representation for and on behalf of midwives.

(Source: The Royal College of Midwives)

The National Childbirth Trust (NCT)
The National Childbirth Trust was formed in 1956 by Prunella Briance, who wanted to promote a more sensitive, woman-centred approach to birth. She followed the philosophy of a doctor called Grantly Dick-Read, who practised in London in the early part of the twentieth century. He believed that childbirth did not have to be a painful and frightening experience for women and that if they understood about what was happening to their bodies, this would lessen the tension and fear they felt while giving birth, and lead to a more fulfilling and empowering experience.

The NCT is a charitable organisation with nearly 70,000 members. It campaigns to improve maternity care, services and facilities for women during childbirth. It offers information and support to women and their partners during pregnancy, childbirth and the early days of parenthood, and runs antenatal classes and postnatal drop-ins for women, and conferences and training for health professionals. In the future the NCT would like to see more women giving birth at home and in birth centres and fewer women giving birth in hospital. It would like to see more support for women to breastfeed and more information about the health benefits of breastfeeding for both mother and baby. Anyone is free to join the NCT – for more information, see www.nct.org.uk.

(Source: The National Childbirth Trust)

CONCLUSION

You should now have a good idea of what nurses and midwives actually do and where they work. If you think this could be the career for you then turn to the next chapter where you can discover what courses and further educational qualifications are available.

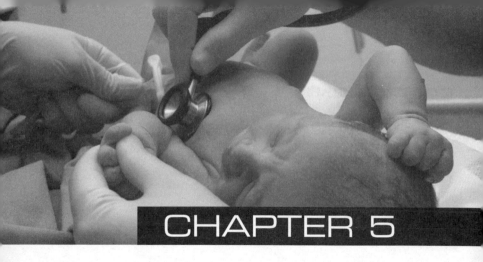

CHAPTER 5

Getting into nursing and midwifery

THE ROUTE TO QUALIFICATION

NURSING

There are four main areas of nursing:

- Adult nursing

- Children's nursing

- Mental health nursing

- Learning disability nursing.

In order to qualify as a registered nurse (RN), you need to take a pre-registration degree or diploma (DipHE) course in nursing leading to registration with the Nursing and Midwifery Council (NMC). Courses usually last three years – the first year will introduce you to all areas of nursing, and in subsequent years you will focus on the particular branch of nursing you have chosen.

MIDWIFERY

In order to qualify as a registered midwife (RM), you need to take a pre-registration degree or diploma course in midwifery leading to registration with the Nursing and Midwifery Council (NMC). Courses usually last for three years and students learn the theory and practice of midwifery in hospitals and in the community. It is possible to 'top up' from a diploma level to a degree at some institutions. Advanced Diplomas are also available, which give more credits at level 3, meaning you can top up to degree level faster.

To find out which courses are available, visit www.ucas.com and www.nmas.ac.uk.

SHORTENED COURSES

Some institutions run shortened courses for nurses who are already qualified and registered and have the relevant experience (ie for those who have a nursing degree/diploma plus six months' practise prior to starting the course). For more information on these courses, please contact the NHS Learning and Development Service on 08000 150 850.

HOW TO APPLY

DIPLOMA COURSES

The **Nursing and Midwifery Admissions Service (NMAS)** processes applications for full-length, diploma-level, pre-registration nursing and midwifery programmes at universities and colleges of higher education in England. However, NMAS does not process applications for degrees in nursing or midwifery, shortened programmes for qualified nurses or midwives, or post-registration programmes.

DEGREE COURSES

The **Universities and Colleges Admissions Service (UCAS)** processes applications for full-time undergraduate degree courses at UK universities and colleges. Further information can be found on their website: www.ucas.ac.uk.

ENTRY REQUIREMENTS

There are no national minimum entry requirements to enter nursing or midwifery courses, as each institution offering a course sets its own criteria. However, all applicants must be able to demonstrate evidence of literacy, numeracy and good character and, in general:

● For a **Diploma programme** most institutions will ask for five GCSEs or equivalent at grade C or above including English language or literature, and a science subject

● For an **Advanced diploma programme** most institutions will ask for five GCSEs or equivalent at grade C or above (including English and a science subject) and two A levels or equivalent

● For a **Degree programme** most institutions will ask for five GCSEs (including English and a science subject) plus two A levels, at higher grades than those required for the Advanced diploma programme.

VOCATIONAL QUALIFICATIONS

The NHS and education sector encourages applications from people with a wide range of academic and vocational qualifications, so if you have no A levels but you do have a recognised vocational qualification, there are many opportunities for you to train in this sector. You may be able to gain direct entry to a Diploma or Degree course – here are some of the vocational qualifications higher education institutions are likely to be looking for:

- NVQ level 3 or above (both general and occupation-specific)

- NVQ level 2 plus one GCSE at grade A–C or equivalent*

- GNVQ Advanced

- GNVQ Intermediate, plus one GCSE at grade A–C or equivalent*

- SQA and SCOTVEC awards (Scottish).

Alternatively, you may be able to train as a nursing assistant, healthcare assistant or maternity care assistant – you will gain an NVQ level 2 qualification and be given relevant on-the-job training, which may enable you to go on to train as a registered nurse or midwife (see the case study with nursing assistant Maxine Holder-Critchlow who has subsequently gone on to be a student nurse: p. 49–50).

FOR THOSE WITH NO FORMAL QUALIFICATIONS ...

If you don't have any formal qualifications, you can take an Access to Health and Social Care course. They are available as both full- and part-time options and are seen as providing the equivalent of two A levels. Courses usually consist of at least four subjects including anatomy, physiology and study skills. You can get more detailed information from your local further or adult education college or from the UCAS access courses database at www.ucas.ac.uk/access.

ENTRY REQUIREMENTS FOR OVERSEAS STUDENTS

Applicants from outside the UK and Eire are required to provide evidence of maths and English. If in doubt, check with the institutions to which you plan to apply to see if your qualifications will be acceptable for entry onto their nursing or midwifery programme.

For further information about entry to nursing and midwifery, see www.nhscareers.nhs.uk or call the NHS Career Helpline on 0845 606 0655.

---

*Midwifery applicants must also have an English and a science (including mathematics) subject at GCSE grade A–C or equivalent.

OTHER FACTORS AFFECTING ENTRY TO NURSING AND MIDWIFERY

In addition to acquiring the right educational qualifications, you will have to satisfy a number of other criteria in order to start your career in nursing or midwifery. A brief outline of each is given below – see www.nhscareers.nhs.uk for further details.

HEALTH AND DISABILITIES

You will need satisfactory health clearance before you are offered a place on a course and each educational institution has its own policy. If you have a health-related problem, such as mobility or hearing difficulties, you should contact the educational institution to which you intend applying to discuss the matter in confidence.

Further help, advice and support for students with disabilities is available from the National Bureau for Students with Disabilities (SKILL) – see www.skill.org.uk. Full contact details are given in the Resources section at the end of this book (Chapter 9).

CRIMINAL RECORDS

As a nurse or midwife you will be in a position of responsibility for vulnerable people. You must therefore declare any criminal convictions you have. Driving convictions of three or more points on your license will also count as a criminal conviction, so these should be declared. Having a criminal record does not automatically prevent you from obtaining a place on a course, but failure to disclose a conviction can result in the withdrawal of an offer, termination of your programme, or disciplinary action.

If you have regular, substantial, unsupervised access to children (which is likely if you would like to work as a nursery nurse, paediatric nurse or midwife), you will have to undergo a **CRB check** to ascertain your full criminal history and to get CRB clearance.

AGE

The minimum age for applicants into nursing and midwifery is 17½ years old at the time when the course begins. For diploma courses, applicants must be at least 16 years old when they apply. There is no upper age limit set by law, and although some universities may set their own limits, most institutions welcome applications from mature candidates.

VISA REQUIREMENTS

If you are not a national of one of the member states of the European Economic Area (EEA) you may need a student visa to study in England. Be aware that a student visa does not enable you to work in the UK after qualification. Make sure you apply for a prospective student entry clearance before travelling to the UK. You'll also need to check your eligibility for financial support with the institution at which you plan to study. For further advice about immigration matters, get in touch with the British Embassy in your country or, if you live in the UK, contact the Immigration & Nationality Directorate – www.ind.homeoffice.gov.uk/ 0870 606 7766.

DOING SOMETHING DIFFERENT – COURSES IN TROPICAL MEDICINE

A course in Tropical Medicine is often valuable for those wishing to work overseas, and may be a requirement for nursing in developing countries. The London School of Hygiene and Tropical Medicine offers the Diploma in Tropical Nursing, which runs twice a year from March to July and from September to February. The course is one day per week and lasts for 19 weeks. It is available to registered nurses only.

The content includes emergency midwifery, dentistry, water and sanitation technology and mental health in the developing world, together with wide coverage of clinical tropical medicine and primary healthcare. Practical skills and laboratory work are also included. For more information, contact the London School of Hygiene and Tropical Medicine on 020 7927 2627 or visit their website, www.lshtm.ac.uk.

(Source: The London School of Hygiene and Tropical Medicine)

FEES AND FINANCE

TUITION FEES

Eligible students finishing NHS-funded degree and diploma courses in nursing or midwifery from 2006/07 will have their tuition fees met in full from the beginning of their course. However you are strongly advised to confirm details of financial arrangements with the NHS Student Grants Unit (www.nhsstudentgrants.co.uk) and with universities before you apply. Overseas applicants will be subject to current residential requirements. For more information visit the Student Grants Unit website: www.nhsstudentgrants.co.uk.

BURSARIES
An NHS bursary is an allowance awarded to eligible students to cover everyday living costs such as accommodation. There are certain criteria applicants must fulfil in order to be eligible for a bursary (such as your residential status) – to find out more, visit www.nhsstudentgrants.co.uk. Funding arrangements for diploma and degree students are different.

DIPLOMA STUDENTS
Funding arrangements for students on NHS-funded nursing or midwifery diploma courses are via an NHS non-means tested bursary. This provides a flat-rate, basic maintenance grant, and no contribution is required from your own income or that of your family. The basic rate is set on the assumption you will be required to attend your course for 45 weeks a year, and varies depending on where you live and where your course is based. In 2005/06, the bursary rate was £6859 for residing in London and £5837 for those living elsewhere or living in their parents' home. If you have to move to London to attend a practice placement, your basic maintenance grant will be temporarily increased by £17 a week. You will also be eligible for a one-off payment of £55, made at the start of the course.

Students receiving the NHS non-means tested bursary are *not* entitled to claim:

- Student loans

- Disabled students' allowance (DSA)

- Access funding

- Hardship loans

- NHS hardship grants.

However, they may be entitled to additional bursaries – see opposite.

DEGREE STUDENTS

Funding arrangements for students on NHS-funded nursing or midwifery degree courses are via an NHS means-tested bursary. This means that your income (or that of your spouse/parents) will be taken into account, and the amount of the grant will be reduced in proportion to that income. Those claiming an NHS means-tested bursary may also be entitled to apply for a Student Loan through their Local Education Authority (LEA).

ADDITIONAL BURSARIES

On top of the bursaries outlined above, there are several categories of additional allowances available as extra payments. This support is available in the following categories:

● Care leavers

● Childcare

● Dependants

● Disabled

● Hardship

● Older students

● Practice placement expenses

● Single parents

● Two homes grants.

Only students in receipt of a NHS student bursary in England and Wales are eligible to apply for any of the additional allowances.

FURTHER INFORMATION ON FUNDING

Contact details of the relevant organisations for England, Northern Ireland, Scotland and Wales are provided in the Resources section at the back of this book (Chapter 9). The website www.nhsstudentgrants.co.uk has detailed information, and a downloadable leaflet *Financial Help for Health Care Students*. You should also contact the institutions to which you have applied.

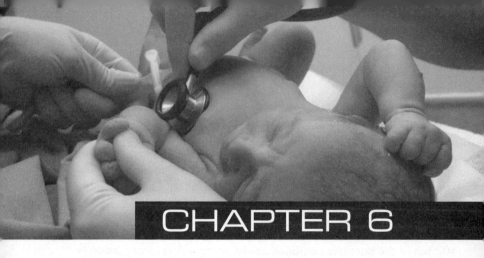

CHAPTER 6

Complementary therapies in nursing and midwifery

According to the BBC, one in five of the population now uses complementary medicine and, with over 50,000 practitioners in the UK working in an industry worth £1.6 billion per year, complementary therapies are an important part of the health sector. This chapter will give a brief overview of the sector and how it can be applied to nursing and midwifery.

WHAT IS COMPLEMENTARY THERAPY?

The *Oxford English Dictionary* defines complementary medicine as 'any of a range of medical therapies not regarded as orthodox by the medical profession'. These days many of us will not only have been treated with conventional Western medicine, but will also have experienced some form of complementary medicine as well. Although complementary therapies should not be seen as an alternative to orthodox medicine, they can add valuable support that recognises the emotional and spiritual well-being of the patient, as well as the physical aspects of healing.

Nowadays, the most commonly used therapies available within the NHS are acupuncture, aromatherapy, chiropractic, homoeopathy, hypnotherapy and osteopathy. A brief outline of each is given below.

ACUPUNCTURE
The origins of acupuncture lie in traditional Chinese philosophy, which states that health is dependent on the body's motivating energy – known as Qi – moving in a smooth and balanced way through a series of meridians (channels) beneath the skin. Qi consists of equal and opposite qualities – Yin and Yang – and when these become unbalanced or blocked, illness may result. Acupuncturists insert fine needles into the channels of energy to stimulate the body's own healing response and help restore its natural balance. You can find acupuncturists working in pain clinics, maternity units and physiotherapy clinics, as well as in their own practices. The World Health Organisation (WHO) has compiled a list of conditions which are appropriate for treatment by acupuncture, including respiratory system problems, the mouth and throat, and neurological and musculo-skeletal disorders.

AROMATHERAPY AND MASSAGE
Aromatherapy is probably the best-known and most widely used of all the complementary therapies. It uses the essential oils from plants combined with massage to promote relaxation and healing in patients with such conditions as insomnia, depression and anxiety. In her book *Aromatherapy: A Nurses' Guide* (Amberwood Publishing Ltd, 1995), Ann Percival states that the benefits of aromatherapy and massage include improving the circulation, stimulating the immune system, reducing muscle tension and revitalising energy levels. Aromatherapy oils you may have in your medicine cabinet include lavender, chamomile and tea tree.

Massage is the art of touch, and involves using the hands to perform movements on the skin to promote relaxation, healing and well-being. The main techniques of Western massage involve stroking, kneading, rubbing or pressing on the body. Aromatherapy massage has been used on cancer patients and those with AIDS and is popular with midwives, although some oils cannot be used during pregnancy because of their potency.

CHIROPRACTIC

Chiropractic means 'done by hand' and involves manually manipulating the body, especially the spine. As the spine protects a large part of the central nervous system, any misalignment or injury to it can affect the nervous system and lead to problems elsewhere. It consists of a wide range of manipulative techniques designed to improve the function of the joints, relieve pain and avoid muscle spasm. Those who most benefit from this treatment include people with lower back pain, migraine sufferers, those with rheumatism and those with sports injuries.

HOMEOPATHY

Homeopathic remedies are based on the theory of 'like treating like' – patients are given very diluted substances that cause the same symptoms as their illness and, in the process, are healed. Homeopathy is used to treat everything from acute fevers, sore throats and toothache to chronic illnesses such as arthritis, eczema, asthma, anxiety and insomnia. It can be prescribed on the NHS and there are a number of hospitals across the UK providing homeopathic treatment.

HYPNOTHERAPY

In hypnotherapy, a therapist induces a trance-like state in the patient making them more relaxed and compliant. It has been used with great success in dentistry on patients who are afraid of dental treatment and some people have even had surgical operations without anaesthetic while hypnotised. It has also been used to help smokers break their addiction to nicotine and some women use self-hypnosis as pain control during labour.

OSTEOPATHY

Like chiropractic, osteopathy is a manipulative technique to diagnose and treat problems with the biomechanical structure of the body. The practitioner uses his or her hands to realign the structural system of the body, relax muscles and improve circulation. About half of the patients who visit osteopaths do so for the treatment of back pain. Other conditions it is used to treat include arthritis, sciatica, sports injuries and rheumatic conditions.

FASCINATING FACTS

In December 1991, the General Medical Council ruled that any GP could employ a complementary therapist to offer treatment on the NHS, as long as the doctor retained clinical responsibility and accountability. However, most of this provision is still outside the NHS, with well over 90% of complementary therapies purchased privately.

(Source: Department of Health press release, 3 December 1991; *Hansard 200*, 3 December 1991; www.bbc.co.uk)

DOES IT WORK?

Although there is still controversy surrounding certain complementary therapies, many have now been recognised as having real health benefits for conditions ranging from allergies to asthma and skin conditions such as eczema. There is an increasing trend towards integrated healthcare where both conventional and complementary therapies are used to benefit the patient. Not only can they work effectively together, but they also provide the patient with a greater sense of control over their own healthcare.

FASCINATING FACTS

According to a report in *Which?* magazine, 82% of people who had had osteopathy said it had cured their problem or made it bearable.

In April 2002 the Royal London Homeopathic Hospital (RLHH), the leading centre for complementary medicine in the NHS, merged with University College London Hospitals NHS Trust (UCLH), showing just how far integration between Western medicine and complementary therapies had come. At Hammersmith Hospitals Trust there is also combined provision of conventional and complementary services in cancer services, and also at the Glastonbury Health Centre complementary medicine service.

Various authorities and watchdogs are beginning to give some complementary therapies a cautious welcome, emphasising that they should be used alongside rather than instead of orthodox medicine. For example, the National Institute for Clinical Excellence (NICE) has backed the use of some complementary therapies in the treatment of multiple sclerosis (MS), saying that doctors should let patients know about the possible benefits of t'ai chi, magnetic field therapy, massage and reflexology. However, many other popular treatments, including acupuncture, yoga, herbal remedies and aromatherapy, have failed to win NICE recognition. NICE also says that, whatever therapy patients choose to pursue, they should be encouraged to tell their doctors about it.

FIRST PROFESSOR OF COMPLEMENTARY THERAPIES IN EUROPE
Europe now has its first professor of complementary therapies in the shape of Professor Edzard Ernst based at Peninsula Medical School in Exeter. The Rufford Maurice Laing Foundation funds his chair allowing him to conduct rigorous, interdisciplinary and international collaborative research into the efficacy, safety and costs of complementary therapies. His department also publishes a review journal called *Focus on Alternative and Complementary Therapies (FACT)*, which aims to present the evidence on complementary therapies in an analytical and impartial manner.

(Source: www.pms.ac.uk/compmed)

HOW DOES COMPLEMENTARY MEDICINE FIT INTO NURSING AND MIDWIFERY?

As complementary therapies become more integrated with mainstream orthodox medicine, knowledge of this area of healthcare will become increasingly useful in order that nurses and midwives are aware of the choices that their patients may make, especially in areas such as palliative care, where complementary therapies are particularly useful. The Nursing & Midwifery Council's (NMC) advice sheet on complementary medicine states that:

'Complementary and alternative therapies are increasingly used in the treatment of patients. Registrants who practise the use of such therapies must have successfully undertaken training and be competent in their area. The appropriateness of the therapy to both the condition of the patients and any co-existing treatments must be considered. It is essential that the patient has been made aware of the therapy and gives informed consent.'

Its Statement of Professional Conduct adds that nurses and midwives must:

'ensure that the use of complementary or alternative therapies is sage and in the interests of patients and clients. This must be discussed with the team as part of the therapeutic process and the patient or client must consent to their use.'

However, in response to a call to include aspects of complementary and alternative medicine (CAM) in the undergraduate nursing curriculum, the Royal College of Nursing recently commented that 'we have no expectation that training in the use of any CAM therapy should be a standard part of a nurse's undergraduate training and would therefore expect that nurses who wish to practise CAM therapies would take up such training post-registration'. So increasingly, nurses and midwives with an interest in CAM therapies will be able to specialise once they have completed their initial RN or RM training.

If you are interested in finding out more, take a look at the *Complementary Therapies in Nursing and Midwifery* journal, which integrates complementary therapies into conventional nursing practices. It covers aromatherapy, massage, acupuncture, reflexology and herbal medicine and features original research, educational issues, best practice reports and book reviews. It is published quarterly by www.harcourt-international.com/journals/ctnm. You will find the names and addresses of the governing bodies for the main complementary therapies in the Resources section of this book (Chapter 9).

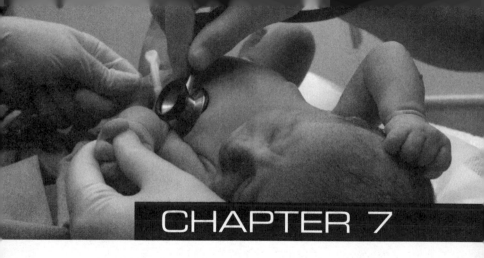

CHAPTER 7

Returning to nursing, midwifery and health visiting

Healthcare professionals are actively encouraged to return to the sector. It doesn't matter how long ago you left – you can still make a significant difference to people's lives. The technological changes in the healthcare sector are only skin deep – the training, expertise and experience you have are still extremely valuable.

For those who are feeling a little rusty, refresher courses can soon update both knowledge and skills. As the NHS careers website states:

'much that has changed in the NHS recently is intended to improve working lives within this vast organisation. There's a greater emphasis on teamwork – so old professional boundaries have been removed in order to deliver more seamless care. In many areas, there's a drive to increase flexibility in working hours, so it's easier to combine work with other commitments. There's more support for staff, and there are more opportunities to develop and acquire new skills.'

It's not only the healthcare sector that has changed; returning nurses, midwives and health visitors tend to be older, wiser, and have more scope in the choices they make. This extra experience and understanding are of real value in their work. If you are thinking of returning to nursing or midwifery, you can expect:

● To be mentored and supported

● To have a named supervisor

● To have flexible patterns of work

● To be supernumerary on your clinical placement

● To have a challenging yet satisfying career.

CASE STUDY – RETURNING HEALTH VISITOR

'What I learned while I was away has enriched the quality of the work I do now,' says returning health visitor Ruth Chorley after an absence of 14 years spent raising a family and working in primary healthcare in Tanzania and Uganda. She says the experience has given her a greater understanding of issues affecting people's health, reaching across cultural and social boundaries. Although what Ruth and her fellow health visitors do has not really changed, she finds that there is now more respect for different races and cultures.

Ruth found a returner's course that she could access from her home near Manchester. Through contact with the Community Practitioners and Health Visitors Association (CPHVA) she joined a six-month part-time course which consisted of three separate weeks of group work in London, coursework she could do at home and shadowing staff in nearby Trusts. The costs of the course were paid by her local consortium. Her persistence paid off when she secured a health visitor post she enjoys, within reach of home.

RETURNING TO LEARNING

New practice requirements mean that nurses, midwives and health visitors who are returners after a gap are likely to have to complete a Return to Practice course in nursing, midwifery or health visiting before starting a job.

If you were previously an Enrolled Nurse, you can convert to become a Registered Nurse by taking a Return to Practice course, starting working again and then looking for a place on a conversion course. Alternatively, you could try for a direct entry conversion course, which would satisfy the return to practice requirement and where you will be eligible for a bursary.

During your Return to Practice course you may be able to choose clinical placements in areas that interest you, and then try to get a job in the area you like most. Once working in this area you can then be supported through an appropriate course. After your course, you will be eligible to join the local bank offering part-time work on a flexible basis, or you may find that you get a job on the ward or unit where you did your clinical placements.

For more information on returning to work in the NHS, contact your local Workforce Development Confederation/Strategic Health Authority, who should have a dedicated return to practice (RTP) coordinator you can talk to, who should also be able to advise you on financial support (see opposite). Alternatively, you can call NHS Careers on 0845 606 0655.

Return to practice courses are offered by local higher education providers and also by distance learning – for example, the Department of Health has funded the production of a distance-learning programme by the Royal College of Midwives (RCM) and the Open University, which is now being run by the RCM and Sheffield Hallam University. Think about what mode of learning is best-suited to your needs.

If you're thinking of returning to nursing in the private sector, BUPA offers a Return to Practice which enables you to renew your registration with the Nursing and Midwifery Council. The programme aims to provide you with the relevant competencies and the opportunity to update and expand your existing skills, giving you confidence in maintaining effective professional care. You will be sponsored by BUPA Hospitals, in partnership with your local university, to undertake a theoretical and practice-based module.

FINANCIAL CONSIDERATIONS

If the thought of the retraining costs is putting you off, don't panic! Assistance with fees is often available (depending on arrangements with your possible employer). Financial support may include a bursary while taking the course, payment for the clinical placement periods of the course and financial assistance with travel costs, books and childcare. Many Return to Practice courses are part-time, enabling you to work while training.

If you go straight into paid employment, your employer will pay you during the retraining period. You may still be eligible for help with travel, books and childcare costs incurred for any external training courses, but will need to confirm this with your local RTP coordinator.

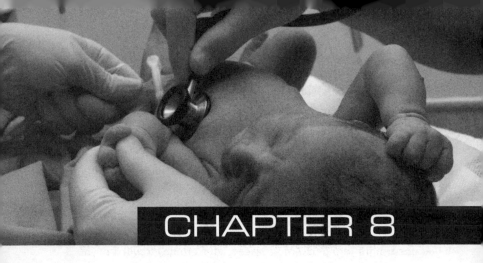

CHAPTER 8

So what's your next move?

Having got this far through the book you should now have a much clearer idea of what working in nursing and midwifery is all about. If you still think this is the career for you (or, if you are a returner, that this is something you really still want to do) then this final section outlines the key questions to ask yourself in order to find out exactly what it is you want to do. You should find that you now have the information you need to come to an informed decision on each point.

AS A NURSE

- Do I want to work in the public (NHS) sector or the private sector?

- Which of the four main sectors of nursing (adult, child, mental health and learning disability) do I wish to work in?

- Do I want to work in a large institution (such as a hospital) or in something smaller within the community?

- Am I satisfied to stay at entry level, or am I ambitious enough to want to climb the promotional ladder?

- Do I want this to be a job for life or the springboard into a laterally connected career?

- Finally, do I really have the strengths and resilience to do this job to the best of my ability?

AS A MIDWIFE

- Do I want to work in the public (NHS) sector, in the private sector (eg as a midwife in a BUPA hospital), or do I want to become an independent midwife (ie self-employed)?

- Could I take on the added responsibility of being a midwife supervisor?

- Do I want to do this because it is a job working with babies, or because I really care for women's welfare and really like women? (If the answer is 'I want to work with babies' then you might be advised to consider a career in nursery nursing or childcare rather than midwifery)

- Finally, do I have the strengths and resilience to do this job to the best of my ability?

You may find it useful to refine your ideas by further research – try talking to people already working in the healthcare sector and, if possible, arrange some work experience so you can work out what it's really like.

GO FOR IT!

Working within the healthcare services can be one of the most rewarding jobs on the planet; saving lives, returning people to full health, restoring their dignity and allowing them to get on with their everyday existence. However, such jobs carry a heavy weight of responsibility and along with the joy can come real pain – when patients die, or you know they will never leave hospital fully restored to health.

The long hours and shifts at night and over the weekends can also drain energy levels and dampen your spirits, so this is not a decision to take lightly. But if you've got the guts, the stamina, the positive attitude, the determination and the vocational calling to be a nurse or a midwife you will find yourself to be a very valued member of society. People really appreciate what you do for them, their families, their friends and for the community at large. If you decide this is really for you then well done – now it's time to go for it! In the next chapter you will find contact details of the organisations you will need to get in touch with to begin your journey to becoming a qualified nurse or midwife.

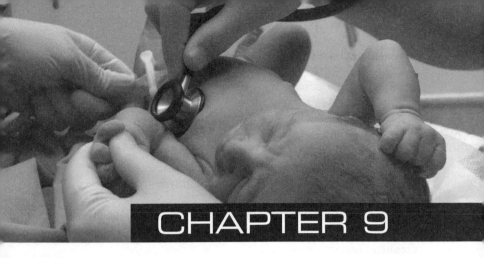

CHAPTER 9

Resources

There is now a wealth of information about nursing and midwifery on the internet and the addresses printed below will give you a more comprehensive view about certain jobs and areas within the sector than we can give in this book.

CAREERS AND TRAINING

- www.independent.co.uk/graduate-options

- www.learndirect-advice.co.uk

- www.ucas.ac.uk

GENERAL NURSING AND MIDWIFERY

Nursing and Midwifery Council (NMC)
23 Portland Place
London W1B 1PZ
Tel: 020 7637 7181
Website: www.nmc-uk.org

UNISON
Tel: 0845 355 0845
Website: www.unison.org.uk
UNISON is the trade union for people working in the health sector.

THE NHS

The following NHS websites are excellent resources packed with everything you need to know about a job within this vast organisation:

- www.careers.nhs.uk

- www.nhs.uk/england/aboutthenhs

- www.institute.nhs.uk

- www.nhsstudentgrants.co.uk

For specific information about particular jobs email advice@nhscareers.nhs.uk.

NURSING

- **Community Practitioners' and Health Visitors' Association**: www.amicus-cphva.org

- **Macmillan nursing**: www.macmillan.org.uk

- **Marie Curie nursing**: www.mariecurie.org.uk

- **Royal College of Nursing (RCN)**: www.rcn.org.uk / 020 7312 3333

MIDWIFERY

- **Independent Midwives Association (IMA)**: www.independentmidwives.org.uk / 01483 821104

- **Midwives Online**: www.midwivesonline.com

- **National Childbirth Trust**: www.nct.org.uk / www.nctresources.co.uk (includes materials for midwives and student midwives)

- **Royal College of Midwives (RCM)**: www.rcm.org.uk / 020 7312 3535

THE ARMED FORCES

- www.armyjobs.mod.uk

- www.rafcareers.com

- www.royal-navy.mod.uk

TRAINING AND EDUCATION

Nursing and Midwifery Admissions Service (NMAS) and Universities and Colleges Admissions Service (UCAS)
Rosehill
New Barn Lane
Cheltenham
Gloucestershire GL52 3LZ
Tel: 0870 112 2200 (applications); 0870 112 2206 (general enquiries)
Website: www.nmas.ac.uk and www.ucas.com

BURSARY SCHEMES

England
NHS Student Grants Unit
NHS Pensions Agency
200–220 Broadway
Fleetwood
Lancashire FY7 8SS
Website: www.nhsstudentgrants.co.uk

Wales
NHS Wales Students Awards Unit
2nd Floor Golate House
101 St Mary Street
Cardiff CF10 1DX

NHS Cymru Uned Dyfarniadau Myfyrwyr
2il Lawr Ty Golate
101 Heol Eglwys Fair
Caerdydd CF10 1DX
Tel: 029 2026 1495
Website: www.wales.nhs.uk

Scotland
The Students Awards Agency for Scotland
3 Redheughs Rigg
South Gyle
Edinburgh EH12 9HH
Tel: 0131 4768212
Website: www.saas.gov.uk

Northern Ireland
The Department for Employment and Learning
Student Support Branch
4th Floor Adelaide House
39–49 Adelaide Street
Belfast BT2 8FD
Tel: 028 9025 7777
Website: www.delni.gov.uk

DISABLED STUDENTS

SKILL Information Service
Tel: 0800 328 5050 (freephone) or 020 7657 2337
Text-Freetext: 0800 068 2422
Website: www.skill.org.uk
Promotes opportunities for young people and adults with any kind of disability in post-16 education, training and employment across the UK.

COMPLEMENTARY THERAPIES

ACUPUNCTURE
- **British Acupuncture Council (BacC)**: www.acupuncture.org.uk

- **British Medical Acupuncture Society (BMAS)**: www.medical-acupuncture.co.uk

AROMATHERAPY
- **Aromatherapy and Allied Practitioners' Association (AAPA)**: www.aromatherapyuk.net

CHIROPRACTIC
- **General Chiropractic Council**: www.gcc-uk.org (the statutory body for Chiropractors)

HOMEOPATHY
- **Society of Homeopaths**: www.homeopathy-soh.org

HYPNOTHERAPY
- **British Society for Clinical Hypnosis**: www.bsch.org.uk

- **National Council for Hypnotherapy**: www.hypnotherapy.org.uk

PUBLICATIONS

- *Complementary Therapies In Nursing and Midwifery* – magazine published four times a year by Harcourt International. Includes reviews and best practise reports

- *Careers in Nursing and Related Professions* by Linda Nazarko. Published by Kogan Page (1997)

- *The Directory of Nursing and Midwifery Courses*, published by Trotman (2005)